Fundamentals of Artistic Therapy

Fundamentals of Artistic Therapy

FOUNDED UPON SPIRITUAL SCIENCE

The Nature and Task of Painting Therapy

DR MARGARETHE HAUSCHKA

Rudolf Steiner Press

LONDON

First published (in German) 1978
First published in English 1985

Translation by Vera Taberner, Anne L. Blathwayt and Ilse H. Ketzel

Publication in English made in agreement with the Schule für
Therapie und Massage, 7325 Boll über Göppingen,
Gruibinger Strasse 29, West Germany.

©1985 Rudolf Steiner Press

ISBN 0 85440 434 1

Printed in Western Germany
by Karl Ulrich & Co, Nürnberg

Contents

Foreword

A medical doctor who had the good fortune to meet Rudolf Steiner and Dr Ita Wegman during her life, and who was able to see for herself the cupola paintings in the first Goetheanum, has caught the spiritual impulse and has used it as the inspiration for her own life's task.

Dr Margarethe Hauschka allowed the impulse which was brought to birth by Ita Wegman, with stimulation from Rudolf Steiner's indications, to flow into her own work and life experience, and through a life-long activity has laid the foundations of a new therapy. She was indefatigable in giving courses at home and abroad, with the purpose of helping this new vocation to come into being, until finally the School for Artistic Therapy (in Boll, Germany) could be founded. Through this possibility for training, she has given her students a set of tools with which they can work independently and fruitfully within this vocation.

Dr Hauschka now offers us an unusual book. It is a continuation of earlier articles which appeared in book form in 1971 on the theme of artistic therapy. In so far as we wish to be fellow participants, she leads us, from out of her own practical experience, objectively but with enthusiasm into the new area of work which she created—in particular during the last fifteen years or so of the School's development.

From her medical, artistic, therapeutic and anthroposophical experience, she gives a concentrated, clearly-formed foundation, which the therapist needs in order that he may ever and again immerse himself in the spiritual basis from which his work springs.

Not only is the essence of artistic therapy and its place within spiritual-scientific medicine described, but a survey is made of the possibilities which stand as principles to the therapist in his area of work. Above all, the bases for judgments are established in such a way that, in the combining of the artistic and medical aspects, the therapeutic aspects shine forth and can be 'read' from the patients. Finally, when everything is taken into consideration, there shines out the essential difference—often too little noticed—between an artistic and a purposeful therapeutic activity.

Artistic therapy is a path of development, a life-long path of training which is not easy. To the many therapists already active, and to all who wish to become so, may the present book be a continually revitalising adviser and helper.

Dr Charlotte Fiechter
4 June 1978

Formative Process

When in 1925 I came for the first time to the 'Klinisch-Therapeutische-Institut' in Arlesheim in order to learn about the curative eurythmy, painting was already taking place with some of the patients. Two artists from Stuttgart, Sophie Bauer and Maria Kleiner, were from time to time commissioned to do this. Both had been active for a period of time in the Goetheanum, helping with eurythmy and other matters behind the stage, and carrying out many errands for Rudolf Steiner. They were close friends, and one might say that they were 'born' therapists. The first indications for painting originated, so far as I know, in the consultation sessions which Dr Ita Wegmann held jointly with Rudolf Steiner. After I had worked with Dr Friedrich Husemann from the summer of 1925 to the autumn of 1927 (he took me as a co-worker because of my knowledge of curative eurythmy), I returned to the Klinisch-Therapeutische-Institut. While with Dr Husemann in Günterstal, I was already able to use simple painting and modelling exercises with the patients, and then continued this in an extended way in my new working situation. Ita Wegman sent me to the branch of the Clinic in the Tessine until 1929; this was at that time not yet in Ascona, but in the Villa Solari on the Lake of Lugano. In these attractive surroundings, and with the task of caring for a limited number of patients both medically and culturally, I had a good opportunity to foster the artistic in many different ways. Eurythmy, painting, drawing, and art excursions into Italy, as well as theoretical studies, belonged to the inner life of this otherwise rather isolated house in Figino, a tiny village on the Bay of Agno.

In 1929 I returned to the Clinic, and found myself involved not only in medical duties but also in looking after the Nurses' Training School which had in the meantime come into being, and which gave yearly courses. I took over the artistic tuition as well as many other subjects connected with the anthroposophical study of man. Ita Wegman arranged matters so that all the co-workers could take part in the artistic activities. She was deeply convinced and expressed this strongly—that the artistic must unquestionably penetrate therapeutic work in just the same way that Rudolf Steiner demanded it should penetrate Waldorf School education. The specific artistic healing could almost unfold of itself during the year of instruction, and in the daily practice with patients. By this is meant, that the daily experiences with the patients proved to be the best tutor.

No curative painting course was given by Rudolf Steiner. Although the conversion of artistic eurythmy into curative eurythmy has always been a pattern for me, one must nevertheless take into consideration that in painting, one is on a quite different level. Curative eurythmy has its fixed exercises and indications. Quite other laws are valid for stimulating the creative forces in painting; one must proceed from the psychic. The psychic disposition of the patient is the inspiration of the therapeutic fantasy from out of which the task is set. Here, fixed tasks would certainly quickly become dead. Yet it is nevertheless necessary methodically to reccognise and learn how the soul forces can be guided in the direction of healing by means of the colours and by the way in which the colours are handled.

The pictures used for illustration purposes (see end of book) consciously avoid the tendency to abstraction in modern painting. As little as curative eurythmy has in common with the aims of stage eurythmy, so far does curative painting lie from the problems of modern art. One arrives at one's goal not in the resultant picture, but through the process of its coming into being and the accompanying experiences.

Artistic therapy is a path to be attained by the involvement of both soul and ego. It demands from the therapist life experience, above all the capacity for empathy, and other qualities which are connected with the renunciation of his own personal artistic work. Ita Wegman called curative art 'sacrificed art'. We know from Rudolf Steiner that if the curative eurythmist takes part frequently in stage eurythmy, his own curative work will suffer, and vice versa. With curative painting the contrast is certainly not so strong, and lies more in the 'how' than in the 'what', but nevertheless it quite definitely exists.

So we worked for twelve years in the Clinic within the developing stream of spiritual-scientifically orientated medicine, until the World War temporarily brought these endeavours to an end, and in 1940 Dr Rudolf Hauschka and I moved for the time being to Austria. Twenty-two years were then to pass until, as a result of giving study courses over many years both at home and abroad, and through the activity of a circle of friends, the School for Artistic Therapy and Massage in Boll, near Göppingen, was able to come into being.

The programme of this school slowly evolved; visiting teachers were invited, and the plan of study was time and again broadened out. Gertrud Bender from Stuttgart, a pupil of Max Wolfhügel (who was the gifted art teacher of the first Waldorf School), played a vital part in laying these foundations. While I feel the deepest thankfulness to everyone who contributed to this result, I would like in addition here to express equally warm thanks to those who above all assisted in bringing this book into existence—Dr Charlotte Fiechter, and my co-worker of many years' standing, Irmgard Marbach; the latter also helped in the founding of the School with full personal commitment.

In view of the fact that we cannot give basic artistic training, we have to require, for the special therapeutic training in Boll, not only active experience with patients but also a purely artistic preparation. Obviously a longer training is needed in order to reach a professional standard. Artistic therapy includes

10

fundamentally all the arts. In the Boll school we are dealing only with the fine arts, with painting, drawing and modelling. Because artistic therapy is only at the beginning of its development, yet is a therapy for the future without which it will no longer be possible to manage, it is necessary that the training develops further.

Therefore, without allowing this knowledge at any time to rigidify into hard and fast rules, what follows is offered as a stimulation and orientation in a certain direction. In order that future therapists are able to awaken the Mercury qualities in their therapeutic fantasy, it is necessary ever and again to refresh oneself creatively from Spiritual Science.

The Rainbow

We must not overlook the fact that in describing the spiritual background of artistic therapy, the same facts must be presented from different aspects and with differing connections. There will therefore necessarily be repetition, but seen as a whole this illumines and deepens our understanding.

We have mentioned before that artistic therapy is a pathway through the soul, a therapy concerned with the realisation of soul-spiritual creative forces of the individuality, which are then able to act upon the deeper-lying bodily processes.

It is therefore not without significance for us to remember that the token or sign of the post-Atlantean culture periods, which are concerned with the development of the soul life, is the bow of colour which Noah saw, and out of which he heard Jehovah's voice saying to him:

> 12 ...This is the token of the covenant which I make between me and you and every living creature that is with you, for perpetual generations.
>
> 13 I do set my bow in the cloud, and it shall be for a token of a covenant between me and the earth.
>
> 14 And it shall come to pass, when I bring a cloud over the earth, that the bow shall be seen in the cloud.
>
> 15 And I will remember my covenant, which is between me and you and every living creature of all flesh; and the waters shall no more become a flood to destroy all flesh.
>
> 16 And the bow shall be in the cloud; and I will look upon it, that I may remember the everlasting covenant between God and every living creature of all flesh that is upon the earth.
>
> 17 And God said unto Noah, 'This is the token of the covenant, which I have established between me and all flesh that is upon the earth.'
>
> (Genesis, Ch. 9, vv 12-17)

Rudolf Steiner, who gave us the key to the world of imaginative pictures in the old religious documents, myths and sagas, confirms in his *Occult Science* the true content of this picture.

The Atlantean period before the Great Flood was concerned with the development of the races, and thus with the development of the differing characterisation of the etheric-physical human body. The post-Atlantean culture periods, on the other hand, were concerned with the unfolding of the soul-spiritual, the stage by stage development of consciousness. Somewhat towards the middle of the Atlantean period, when the human being had developed his physical body to the stage of ego-uprightness, the ego began to work inwardly and to develop different parts of the soul. The post-Atlantean culture periods described by Rudolf Steiner are the stages through which the spirit strides forward through time. The ego expands in all directions in a sunlike manner, and so causes an inward-turning process at the same time as outwardly initiating a gradual conquest of the earth through the senses. By means of the breathing, the astral body and ego slowly penetrate ever more deeply into the bodily processes in order stage by stage to activate on the one hand the life of the senses, and on the other, the will life, to ever new capacities.

With the fifth culture period we stand in the middle of this development. How this mirrors itself in the artistic creation of mankind will be dealt with in a later publication. But there are already books on this theme by several students of Rudolf Steiner. A more exact knowledge of these processes belongs to the training of artistic therapists, in order by means of this to gain stimulation for the therapeutic work. The light is the meduim in which the soul-astrality of the cosmos lives. World astrality streams along the light-rays from sun, stars and moon, and is 'World soul' in the air space of the earth, which we breathe in. The human soul is also a being of light, and formerly in Paradise we were light-breathing beings. But when the 'light-soul' had to descend into the darkness of the denser elements, into the etheric-physical body which represents the darkness, so the colour realm came into being as the bridge. Goethe's genius has rediscovered what was known in all the old Mystery Centres, namely, that the colour cosmos is the mediator between the heavenly world of light and the earthly darkness of matter. This process is already described in detail in the first chapter (on Plant Colours) of my small book *Zur Künstlerische Therapie*, and its consequences are also shown. The soul lives in the earth realm in the deeds and sufferings of the light. In the outer rainbow, the World soul reveals itself in its cosmic ordering. The phenomenon of the rainbow in Nature is, for the penetrating observer of this 'parable', a sensible/supersensible experience; for Goethe it was also a sensible/moral experience, for the moral is already supersensible. In the world of colour, the heavenly unites with the earthly world, and the colours hover as yet weightless between spirit and matter as the phenomenon of the middle realm, as Bifrost Bridge—to quote our German forefathers—over which the gods ascend and descend.

Today, we only have knowledge of the physical phenomenon: if the sun is behind us, and a dark wall of cloud in front of us, then the waterdrops to the left and right of our shadow, acting prismatically at an angle of approximately 42°, conjure up the bow of colour before our eyes, beginning with red outside and ending inside with blue-violet. One can also say that the active colours turn towards the outside and the passive inwards, while in between is the luminous green. This is the physical phenomenon, the 'body' of the rainbow, so to speak. The soul's bow of colour, whether it be connected with the feeling life or even with human capacities, has the reversed sequence of colours.

At this point I would like to allow Rudolf Steiner to speak in his own words, where in the fourteenth lecture of the 'Speech and Drama Course' he describes the phenomenon:

I can really tell you nothing that will help you so well to develop a sensitive feeling for stage décor as will the rainbow. Give yourselves up in reverent devotion to the rainbow, and it will develop in you a remarkably true eye for stage-setting, and moreover the inner ability to compose it.

The rainbow!...I feel within me a mood of prayer: that is how the rainbow begins, in the intensest violet, that goes shimmering out and out into immeasurable distances. The violet goes over into blue—the restful, quiet mood of the soul. That again goes over into green. When we look up to the green arc of the rainbow, it is as though our soul were poured out over all the sprouting and blossoming of Nature's world. It is as though, in passing from violet and blue into green, we had come away from the gods to whom we were praying, and now in the green were finding ourselves in a world that opens the door to wonder, opens the door to a sensitive sympathy and antipathy with all that is around us. If you have really drunk in the green of the rainbow, you are already on the way to understanding all the beings and things of the world, Then you pass on to yellow, and in yellow you feel firmly established in yourself, you feel you have the power to be man in the midst of Nature, that is, to be something more than the rest of Nature around you. And when you go over to orange, then you feel your own warmth, the warmth that you carry within you; and at the same time you are made sensible of many a shortcoming in your character, and of good points too. Going on then to red, where the other edge of the rainbow passes once again into the vast distances of Nature, your soul will overflow with joy and exultation, with ardent devotion, and with love to all mankind.

How true it is that men see but the body of the rainbow! The way they look at it is as though you might have an artificial figure of a man in front of you, made of papier-mâché, and were quite content with this completely soulless human form. Even so do men look up at the rainbow, with no eyes or feeling for anything more than that.

When pupils of a dramatic school go for excursions, they should take every opportunity that offers for entering into this living experience of the rainbow. (Naturally, one cannot arrange for such things, but the opportunity comes more often than people imagine.) For it is like this. One who is training for the stage has to come to grips with the earth. In running, leaping, wrestling, in discus-throwing and in spear-throwing—in the practice of these he enters right into the *life of the earth*. He must, however, also find his way, through the heavenly miracle of the rainbow, into a deep inner *soul experience of colour*. Then he will have found the world on two sides, making contact with these two revelations of it. And a *revelation of the world*—that is what drama has to be!

When the student is running, leaping, wrestling, he isn't just executing a

14

movement that he can see; he is *within* the running and the leaping with his *will*. And now, when with the eye of the soul he beholds the colours of the rainbow, he is not looking at Nature merely in her outer aspect, he is face to face with the soul-and-spirit that is in Nature—which is what we must also succeed in bringing on to the stage, for without it our décor will never be truly artistic. Beholding thus the soul-and-spirit that works and weaves in Nature, the student will verily be on the way to becoming a contemplator of the universe, he will be learning frankly and naively to contemplate, in soul and spirit, the great wide universe. And that will mean, he will find his way back again to the little children's verse that one used to hear so often in earlier days:

> *Kind, es kommt der liebe Gott gezogen*
> *Auf einem schönen Regenbogen.*

(Rudolf Steiner, Colour)

(The dear God comes to us, my child,
Upon a lovely rainbow.)

What is expressed here in connection with stage art concerns the painter still more intensively and variedly, and the therapist most deeply of all. Raphael-Mercury, the healing force, acts in the breathing process which must penetrate us right into the last cell. In a similar manner the colours must bring harmonious order into every corner of the sick person's soul, or at least be able to pave the way towards harmony. But our physical-etheric bodies have today become so terrestrially hardened that the effectiveness of this action has already become weakened. We are however moving towards a future when the therapies will become ever more liberated from matter and more spiritual, and when above all the human ego will be stimulated to individual activity; in fact, without the activity of the ego, no real healing will be possible any more.

Whoever wishes to enter deeply into the cosmic-earthly phenomenon of the rainbow and its primal position as mediator between heaven and earth, will find a magnificent summary of all the manifestations in this realm in Dr Walter Bühler's book: *Nordlicht, Blitz und Regenbogen*, published by the 'Philosophisch-Anthroposophischen Verlag' at the Goetheanum. Reference is also made there to the fact that the rainbow is the only phenomenon in Nature which depends for its appearance, not only on sun and earth but also on man himself, for the rainbow itself moves with the observer. 'Each person sees his own separate bow of colour'. Everyone, by reason of the way in which he is placed between heaven and earth, and through the activity of his sense organisation, separates out from the universal Sea of Colour his own individual form—his own rainbow. This is only possible because this Sea of Colour is not a surging chaos, but a well-ordered fabric of flowing colour penetrated by its own inner law. (This description does not apply to lightning or to the Northern Lights.) And then he goes on:

The circle of colours then accompanies us step by step and yet never comes nearer to us. It leaves us free. It therefore becomes evident why the silent majesty of this harmonious wonder, which the sevenfold coloured splendour reveals in balanced rhythms, exerts such a characteristically beneficent fascination on one's feelings. Anyone who cannot open his heart to this is in danger of becoming psychically ill; his place as a balanced human being in relation to the cosmos would be basically endangered.

At this point, the Goethean method of observation already broadens out into the spiritual-scientific study of man. The soul element, the astrality, is indistinguishable from the colours, it lives in them, reveals itself and moves in them. Our feeling life is a surging of colour between thinking in light, and willing which comes into being in the darknessss of the bodily processes. The sun in the cosmos, and the ego in the microcosm, continually organise this surging movement into the breathing harmony of the bow of colour. It is the token of peace, as expressed in a former time by Jehovah. Peace enters the soul if the opposing poles are brought into colour harmony.

The first appearance of the rainbow followed the downfall of Atlantis, which occurred through the betrayal of the Mysteries—that is, through the premature and egoistic use of the Life Forces, which then acted in an untimely way on the Elements. At that time, the human being still possessed the power of imagination, a dreamlike life of pictures, an old astral clairvoyance and sometimes clairaudience. The surroundings were immersed in mist; the remembrance of this emerges in the northern mythology in the picture of Nifelheim. The senses of the people of Atlantis were then more full of life, with softer organs penetrated with warmth, and through the etheric body were connected with and even nourished by the surrounding elements. Pythagoras still called their glance 'a warm exhalation'; and even in the Christian legend of Dietrich, the furious glances of the hero melt the weapons of his opponents. Slowly the eye became deadened to an outer sense organ. The etheric body withdraws and the light penetrates from outside. The sound and life ethers remain more strongly active at the back of the eye. Noah, the initiate of the transition perod, saw the peach-blossom bow— the light born out of darkness—still as an etheric red, but he also still heard the sound impression of the voice of Jehovah. Then in the course of development the imaginative pictures slowly fade away, and on account of this the sense impressions appear brigher and clearer. Out of the etheric red, the ability to see the outer colours slowly comes into being. Albert Steffen has described in earlier writings how, from the beginning of the Old Indian culture until that of Greek times, the yellowish-reddish tones prevailed, the green first appearing shortly before the Turning Point of Time. The ancients first saw the rainbow, as a peach-blossom red arch, the Bifrost Bridge of the Germanic tribes was red, and the red bull stood upon it to protect it. The active colours were the first to be experienced. Only gradually death enters into the life of the senses, causing them to dry up; the imagination is destroyed and at the same time the ability to see outer colours is strengthened. The blue dome of heaven still had, in the experience of the Greeks, an impresson of red, and until the time of Homer there was no word for blue. After the Mystery of Golgotha it gradually became possible to see the pure blue, the 'lustre of the soul'. Many painters give a picture of this incisive experience, as represented by Mary's blue mantle. Today we see the rainbow

16

from indigo to the deepest red as an outer sense perception, but there are no gods ascending and descending, and the bow is silent.

This necessary development accompanies man's path into the darkness of the material world so that he may acquire a free ego-consciousness and a purified force of love out of the organising forces of the earth-will.

As in the macrocosm the divine hierarchies move to and fro over the rainbow bridge between the spiritual world of light and the material world of darkness, so the microcosmic spirit of man moves to and fro between thinking in light and willing in the darkness of the body, always over the rainbow bridge of the middle realm, through our colourful human feeling-life, through that middle realm where, in artistic creation—in the play impulse—Schiller considers that the true man and his eternal entelechy are most clearly revealed. The being of the rainbow is inexhaustible, and God viewed it as a door to mankind's goal. Although the soul is imprisoned in flesh, humanity will not be forgotten. A Christ-prophecy is hidden in this simple sentence, that at some future time the inner rainbow will also resurrect, as is indicated in the aura of the Resurrected One in the picture of the Isenheim Altar.

After all that has been said, it is not surprising that the whole training for colour therapists begins with the rainbow, with the unity of colours in their cosmic ordering, with the pure phenomenon, an ever-repeated meditative observation of which can lead to an inexhaustible source of healing forces.

But the rainbow—the mirror picture of the World soul in the World ether—is not a dead mirror picture but one filled with life: it is the microcosmic image of the Star forces in the Elements, which the Egyptians venerated by the name of Isis. She represents the World astrality which has not gone through the Fall of Man, and is therefore the archetype for the harmony of forces which we call health. As was already described in the first volume,* in the Egyptian Mysteries of healing the soul was brought before Isis in the 'Temple Sleep', so that it might be corrected by the archetype; and later, on awakening, this correction is transmitted to the physical-etheric body. As the vision of Isis became clouded and no longer attainable, the same forces were sought for in a world nearer to the earth, in Nature. Isis became the goddess Natura whom Brunetto Latini in the thirteenth century was once more able to perceive, until she too disappeared from the consciousness of mankind, and the perception of earthly matter remained the only attainable possibility. Kali Yuga, the Age of Darkness, took its course. The Mystery of Golgotha then marks the turning point in mankind's history. With the forces brought by the Christ, a new ascent becomes possible. Now, however, the individual ego, through active work must conquer the way to a new breakthrough to knowledge of the spiritual world and to new methods of healing. The active therapies are the therapies of the future, even if for a long time yet, substance has to be used. But already the founder of Homoeopathy, Hahnemann, shows that in substance itself, through the potentising process which is a process in the direction of dematerialisation, the healing forces can be released in a new way.

*Zum Künstlerischen Therapie, Band I - not yet translated into English.

The Soul's Inner Rainbow

In the previous chapter, in the quotation from the 'Speech and Drama Course' by Rudolf Steiner, the inner rainbow of human soul moods and capacities already began to appear. There are however some still more penetrating descriptions by him. The colours are able to bring the psychic to expression perfectly, as they are the medium in which the astrality lives. The world of colour is itself, like the astrality, organised polarically; what in the psychic constructive world forces are Sympathy and Antipathy, are here in the world of colour, light and darkness. When the astrality plunges in Sympathy into the material body, the will is produced on the basis of the blood. When the astral body frees itself from the restraint of physiological processes, this allows Antipathy to be active in the physical, as happens in the nerves-and-senses system, enabling the physical to act as a mirror for the creation of consciousness, and the possibility of knowledge arises. The soul is able to work in two directions. There is a colour sketch by Rudolf Steiner which clearly shows this relationship. In the rainbow which is 'turned inwards' and completely surrounded by blue, a profile is to be seen looking towards the inner light space where it passes over from green to blue (picture 2). The whole is in this way a picture of our soul space, swimming, so to speak in the blue of the enclosing world soul. Outwardly, our consciousness is limited through our concepts of the Infinite becoming ever more indefinite and abstract, represented by green as the restricting intellectual-soul activity. If however we descend into the depths of our own soul, then through the capacity of memory, which is already strongly connected with the body, we reach, through the red, to the 'blood' side. Thus, seen psychically, we really are, as human beings, such creations of light, formed through the Being of colour in a threefold way. From a middle position we are able to advance on two paths, one outer and one inner, towards the cosmic world forces—here represented by the enclosing blue.

Rudolf Steiner has made use of the speech of colour in different ways, in order that better sketches of the relationships might restore to life—and create a deeper understanding for—certain diagrams; for colour is always able to unlock a new door to knowledge. But one may never say that a specified colour belongs to the subject with which it is linked. Nevertheless the themes of a diagram are in the same relationship to each other as are the colours with which they are characterised. An example may illustrate this. In the lecture—of great importance for every therapist—of 14 February 1920 on the 'Feeling, Desiring and Willing of the Human Being', the upper and lower human soul qualities are represented by colours in the following way: the upper qualities of perception, intelligence and memory in rainbow form, from indigo through dark and light blue to green, yellow, orange, red. So, the intelligence extends from light blue to green, then follow transitions through yellow, orange to red—the colour of the memory, becuase this, as already previously mentioned, must be supported by the bodily processes. To the lower soul qualities of feeling, desire and will are assigned the colours of deep red, red-violet and blue-green. And then follows the hint that, for example, intelligence is related to desire in the same way as light blue-green is related to red-violet; so it becomes a question of the sensible/moral experience which the colours arouse in the soul. These are capable of comparison.

There are indeed very many different colour connections, for example, also to the planets. It is always only a question of which aspect of a many-sided reality will reveal itself in this particular combination. Colour has the capacity for revelation. But in the soul it passes over into a sound experience which lies deeper. Musical laws arise when the ego descends half-a-stage into the astrality. The sun 'resounds' when it traverses the starry heavens in twelve musical keys; this music contains the laws of the spirit in the soul. From this point of view music is a more powerful art which can penetrate the material world as otherwise only warmth—which carries the spirit downwards—is able to do. Consequently there lives within music a magical force which organises matter from within; substance begins to vibrate in the world of sound. In addition, the human being is not able to close himself off from music even though he may be deaf. But colour leaves the human being entirely free. When I look at colour and absorb it, it speaks the language of my soul. But music seizes me with the force of destiny and is able to speak about the experience of my ego on the spiritual path.

Let us return to the inner rainbow. If, through our ego, which is our soul 'sun', we are in equilibrium between our upper and lower forces, then the bow in us is also harmonious, and full of life simply from its own nature so long as the forces continally breathe into each other and everything is united together in a healthy way. In the same way that the outer rainbow appears as a half-circle on the earth, so colour makes use only of the upper human being, despite the fact that it represents the whole human being in his threefoldness. In the nerves and senses system, where the astral body, and partially also the etheric body, are free from the physical basis, we grasp outwards with, so to speak, an invisible limb, take in the pictures of the world and impress them into ourselves. Thereby the blue side of the spectrum is related to the cool head forces—the details will be discussed in the chapter on the single colours—and works therefore in a calming manner from above downwards and does not stimulate the nerves and senses system; thus through the observation of blue, our inner red, bound to the processes of the blood, flows downward from the head. The opposite happens with the observation of red. As a reaction, red lifts the blood processes upwards to the head, which means that the sense organs become rather more livingly penetrated with blood. All this is more noticeable with the animals who have no controlling ego. The bull becomes aggressive through red. The tiger will avoid blue living places. The nervous system and the blood, the upper and lower astral body, stand opposite to one another in a certain tension similar to that of blue and red. In the nerves-and-senses system, the macrocosmic forces penetrate inwards and call forth the answer—the sensible/moral reaction.

Between macrocosm and microcosm lies our skin, which belongs to the nerves-and-senses system and which, by transformation, enables the sense organs to come into being. Each part of the skin could, for example, produce an eye, and the whole of the skin plays an important role in the assimilation of light. There is a law, however, which is valid also for Hydrotherapy. The force which I apply from outside attracts a similar force from within myself to the periphery. In the skin, and more especially in the senses, cosmic and human-microcosmic qualities come to terms with each other, and the colours therefore also call forth the complementary colours. The etheric body answers, and supplements each specific stimulus to a wholeness. So, for example, red calls forth green, which is yellow and blue; blue calls forth orange, which is yellow and red; yellow calls forth violet, which contains red and blue. Colour shows us here nothing but a generally valid law which is able to lead us to a deeper understanding of therapeutic action. The healing forces of Mercury are hidden in the breathing, and breathing already shows the same phenomenon—the destructive in-breathing as an illness-causing characteristic calls forth the out-breathing as its healing solution. The breathing is as it were the pertinent archetype. Here the astral body continually immerses itself half-a-stage into the etheric body and is immediately expelled again. In order to understand better the phenomenon of self-healing in its relation to the causing of illness through the processes of the nerves-and-senses system, I would like to quote some fundamental sentences from the book by Rudolf Steiner and Ita Wegman, *Fundamentals of Therapy*, as follows:

> Even the normal way in which the astral and ego-organisation take hold of the human body, is related not to the healthy processes of life, but to the diseased. Wherever the soul and spirit are at work, they annul the ordinary functioning of the body, transforming it into its opposite. In so doing they bring the body into a line of action where illness tends to set in. In normal life this is regulated directly it arises by a process of self-healing...In the faculties of soul and spirit, therefore, we have to seek the cause of disease. Healing must then consist in loosening this element of soul or spirit from the physical organisation.

This is one way of being ill. But there is another. This other way of being ill will be discussed in what follows.

The self-healing forces are of course situated in the etheric body which, in response to the encroachment of the astral body, again restores the totality, which leads to wholeness and to 'healing'. This corroborates the phenomenon of the complementary colours in the world of colour. One learns the speech of colour only through a meditative deepening of one single colour within the broad

20

compass of the soul. The following descriptions should be regarded as a summary of the various indications given by Rudolf Steiner, which can form a basis for each person's own efforts. To this study the following may be added: one must not forget that there are not only seven but also twelve colours as there are twelve musical keys. We have seen that the musical element arises when the ego slips down half-a-stage deeper into the astrality. In a cosmic sense, this means when the World-ego, the sun, together with all its planets, travels through the starry heavens, through the cosmic astral world, through the twelve signs of the Zodiac; then the Harmony of the Spheres arises out of the infinite variety of the constellations and their movements. If on the other hand the astral body slips down half-a-stage into the etheric body, then painting arises—flowing colour in all its variety.

The seven colours of the rainbow correspond moreover to the curved day path of the sun through the star pictures from the Ram to the Scales. The other five correspond to the might path of the sun from Scorpio to the Fishes, and here the colours are five shades of peach-blossom—a blueish-violet for Scorpio, a reddish colour for the Fishes. In the middle stands Capricorn in a quite neutral peach-blossom. The colours of the veils were designed in this arrangement by Rudolf Steiner for the presentation of the signs of the Zodiac in eurythmy. One can also experience peach-blossom, the colour of the healthy human skin, as a pale 'purpur'. In Goethe's *Theory of Colour*, 'purpur' is the highest intensification and corresponds therefore to the power of the ego, the individuality which brings together a polarity into a unity.

The care and enlivening of this inner rainbow—the movements of the soul in the colour space—today ought to begin for children already in their schooldays, because the soul-destroying forces of excessive intellectuality and materialism can gradually lead to soul blindness. With the over-valuation of intellectual understanding, through which everyone develops only the egoism of his own viewpoint, the tendencies to illness greatly increase.

This characteristic of the world of colours, to breathe by means of the complementary colours, should be emphasised in therapy and lifted into consciousness if one wishes especially to stimulate this process. Then one would also take pictures by Van Gogh, Macke and Marc and other painters which are composed in strong luminous colours with a complementary quality. If one enhances the single colour to its greatest luminosity (for example, in veil painting, but also in other techniques) without it becoming too dense and physical, then the breathing is considerably deepened.

In the quotation from the medical book by Rudolf Steiner and Ita Wegman, it is said at the end that what is described is one way of becoming ill, and that there is yet another way. This other way comes about in an opposite manner. In this case, the higher members, the astral body and the ego, are prevented from making the loose breathing connection with the physical body which normal feeling, thinking and willing bring about. Then a too luxuriant etheric activity sets in, and one must so deal with the etheric body that it again tends to attract the higher members. From the soul aspect one should stimulate the astral body and ego of the sick person to greater activity in order that they may grasp more strongly into the physical.

Various possibilities serve the artistic path—for example, black and white drawing, composition exercises, also copying and other activies which will be mentioned later. One should note well that there are never fixed recipes but only general directions from which the therapeutic fantasy must find the effective remedy for each single situation.

To be sure, in no one today is the inner rainbow so ordered as is the heavenly one. This ordering remains the distant lofty goal which the soul glimpses when it dares to look at it, and remains an ever-repeated reminder to strive after this goal. One may surely say that already today the Divine beings are again coming over the rainbow bridge to the earth. Over the rainbow bridge built by the human ego, the Christ forces are able to enter our hearts and grant to the soul in the turmoil of its destiny, moments of peace—for the rainbow is the Bow of Peace.

The Vocation of the Artistic Therapist

In the previous chapter it was described how, when the situation is a healthy one, our changing moods of soul are experienced in their connection with the body, very little or not at all. The soul is then an instrument for all possible 'musical keys', pictorially expressed, and this instrument is at the same time rightly tuned. But even the idiom of language says that 'being out of tune' accompanies illness or often already announces it, before there is anything to be observed physically. In illness, the harmonious interplay of the members of one's being is disturbed; in particular it is the astral body which stimulates the life processes either too much or too little, and the controlling ego cannot immediately restore the harmony again. Now each artistic exercise stimulates the creative forces of the ego in the most manifold ways. As we have seen, painting arises in the play between the astral and etheric bodies, and on this level the ego becomes active and brings both into a breathing connection through the medium of the colour and the painting. This activity corresponds to a binding together—that is, to a stronger connection —through the in-breathing, and a loosening through the out-breathing. Through the use of active therapy, we come to the assistance of the self-healing forces of the human being, which always, through a stronger ego activity in the middle region of the human being—his inner Mercury—work in many different directions. The story of Baron Münchhausen* reads like a high-spirited fantasy, but it is nevertheless also a picture of how we grasp the astral body—this fantastic Baron—from above and are able to pull ourselves out of the swamp, or, by a stoke of genius, ride through the air on a cannon-ball. The therapist must therefore above all possess a good understanding of the characteristics of the single members of the human being. The development of this faculty is a part of his training, for which, generally speaking, the anthroposophical study of man creates the essential foundation.

The therapist should have convincingly experienced the difference between art and healing art. Every reasonable person knows that great art also contains healing forces for mankind, so long as it fulfills Goethe's demand of making visible the invisible. In a genuine work of art, the spirit must shine through the material form.

*(Note for English readers): German children know and love these stories of the 18th century Baron Münchhausen. In the first story, his horse falling into a swamp, he at once pulled himself out by his own pigtail and then pulled his horse out. In the second, he mounted a flying cannon-ball in order to see into a besieged city. Meeting another cannon-ball coming the other way, he jumped from one to the other in mid air, and so came safely home. (Transl.)

Now in the present-day natural-scientific era, the fall into materialism, and the evaluation of things only from purely earthly-materialistic aspects, bestow great uncertainty on us, not to speak of chaos in the realm of art. A disintegration or cutting into pieces of the form, abstract compositions, the arbitrary action of over-emphasised individualism, all confuse the true feeling for art. So alongside a serious movement in art, which seeks new paths in order to thrust through to the creative forces behind the sense world, there arises much on the other hand which one must call sick. Today art, out of its own nature, does not act unconditionally in a beneficial manner, but in its over-intellectualisation and arbitrary one-sidedness can also produce illness-causing results. Some years ago, a case was mentioned in the paper of a painter in Paris who could only be cured of his heart complaint when he altered his style of painting, and suffered relapses each time he tried to return to his old habits.

There is a great difference between art and healing art in the way it is practised. The artist does everything with the work of art in mind; the curative painter or therapist has the sick person in the centre of his attention. If he has grasped the healing requirement of the patient through the forces of a loving 'feeling into' his soul situation, then he will endeavour to transform this healing requirement into an artistic task. If the patient has need of a stronger in-breathing, a strengthening of his soul and of the connection of his ego with his soul, then one would call on the plastic forming forces (modelling, black-and-white drawing, object drawing and painting, etc.); and in the contrary situation, one would employ the loosening forces of the 'wet' painting technique or similar contour loosening exercises for the out-breathing, and against cramping tendencies. Within this rather concise characterisation there is of course still a wide scope for the artistic-therapeutic fantasy. This has to be especially trained. Therefore the healing art is for the therapist an art which has been 'sacrificed', as Ita Wegman frequently expressed it. He does not work at that which he himself would like to realise artistically, but a selfless 'turning towards' the sick person is the presupposition of the therapy. Compared with the artist, this signifies a swing of 180°. This same swing certainly also arises between stage eurythmy and curative eurythmy. Both demand the involvement of the whole human being.

The personal soul problems of the therapist should never be discussed, and on the whole, the less they come into view, the better. The patient seeks advice and support, and his trust is won by someone who is at peace with himself and who radiates calmness and certainty.

First of all then, the practical experiences will be described which have been made with regard to the outer administration of artistic therapy.

If one works in groups, as is always to be met with in clinics, sanatoria, and therapeutic centres, or in private practice in addition to the individual treatment, a special room should be set aside for this, as is generally customary in such institutions. This room should possess a warm, inviting atmosphere, should contain no glaring colours or pictures, and should look well-cared for. Before the painting session, the place for each patient should be prepared and everything put ready, otherwise he has too little time afterwards to become absorbed in the painting task. The finished pictures may after the session be hung up in order to show progress. This allows each of the participants to have an interesting succession of pictures whose positive features can be discussed, so stimulating further activity; frequently they contain an intimation of the next task. There must if possible be quiet during the session. The therapist himself gives the necessary instructions quietly, and should be able to soften his voice. 'Trumpeters' are no therapists! At the same time there should not be the slightest suggestion of a mystical mood, but only a considerate, relaxed, somewhat cheerful, and above all completely natural atmosphere, which makes it easy for the patients to come out of themselves a little and to experience joy in their artistic endeavours. That is ultimately the most important thing, and everything else should contribute to this aim.

One might think that all this is somewhat self-evident, but experience has shown that the therapeutic instinct—the unconscious knowledge of that which is necessary—begins in many areas to fail in our intellectual time, in fact, to be completely lost.

There is also today, in the choice of a profession, less and less heed or consideration paid to the real suitability of a person, or for what purpose he feels himself 'called' in the deeper sense. It is not the head, nor the intelligence quotient, which determines the good therapist, but the Mercurial qualities of the centre. A separate chapter will be devoted to the working of Mercury, in order to broaden historically where the sources of the healing forces lie, and how men of past cultures strove to reach them. The Mercurial centre should carry the ego, the real kernel of the human being, as the regulating ruler of the soul-life and reveal it in the manner of the conduct of life. The ego is sunlike and forms us into an individual personality. As the real centre point, it creates each moment the balance between the polar forces of the upper organisation, which serves the growth of consciousness, and the lower, which serves the formation of the will through the metabolism. But also between all soul forces, which of course have polar character in that for each quality there exists its opposite, the ego forms the supporting fulcrum of the scales. The upper human being is more strongly permeated with the forces of the ego, and is, since the 'Fall of Man', a fighter against the lower, which contains a stronger animal quality, that is to say, our instincts, desires and passions. In olden times such real facts were always expressed in mythological pictures. For all the representations of the conquering forces of the ego against the animalistic nature point to this: the fight of Mithras with the bull, the fight of Michael or St George with the dragon. They open the eyes of humanity to its task. But we achieve this victory over the lower nature only when the earthly ego unites with the sunlike World Ego, with the Christ, whom the alchemists called the 'Verus Mercurius' so long as they still possessed genuine spiritual wisdom.

The Christ Sun-forces bring the healing to the world, of which each single healing is so to speak a droplet, a copy in miniature. If therefore one wishes to work in the sphere of artistic activity in order to heal, one should possess certain qualities, or at least strive subsequently for those that lie in this direction. Ita

Wegman writes about this in her article *Das Mysertium der Erde*:*

> The Ego of man, the most individual part of man, has the peculiarity not to wish to remain within itself, but to immerse itself in the being of the other. That which one calls base self-seeking is entirely foreign to it.

The true Ego kindles brotherliness in the soul, fellow-feeling, the ability to enter into the other soul, in order in this way to come to know its healing requirement. This signifies taking the way of Parsifal, which is characterised by the words: 'through compassion to come to knowledge'. The point is not to wish to exhibit oneself, but to develop the qualities of the bee and the ant, that is to say, to be able humbly to acquiesce in a higher ordering, to be industrious, to have devotion to the small things in one's conduct, and to develop still other beneficial virtues. The Greeks called the pupil of the Mysteries who had reached a certain grade, a 'Bee'. The ants are those who regularly heal the soil in our woods, and who lead the dying substance back into the life process.

On the other side, this profession demands from the therapist a conscientious training, not a smattering of many things but a fully experienced and ensouled world picture. What is meant is the manner of thinking similar to that which lies at the basis of Goethe's scientific and artistic works, in which living ideas hold sway, a perception of the world which led him to an 'intuitive power of judgement'. When Goethe's gaze rested on a phenomenon, he did not brood upon its meaning. With the constantly repeated perception, the phenomenon finally expressed itself to him; and the force streaming from his 'sunlike' eyes which, if one observes the world lovingly, ascends from the heart into the sense organs, was able with Goethe, to penetrate through the appearance to the living creative forces which the phenomenon had built up from the spiritual side, that is to say, to the archetypal form. The pure sense perception was able to pass over into Imagination. Therefore Goethe said to Schiller, when the latter called the archetypal plant 'only an idea', that he was then happy that he could see his ideas really before his eyes. It is the middle, feeling, human being where the forces of enthusiasm, of an inspired working with all one's might, also of transfiguration and positivity, are at home, which here manifests his slumbering capacities. These soul moods will be carried by the process in the etheric body which Rudolf Steiner describes as the 'etherisation of the blood'. The etherisation-stream in the blood moving from the heart upwards is able again to enliven to living picures the dead thoughts in the head, as a first step to genuine Imagination. Without mobilising the forces of the heart, one is not able to arrive at an intuition of the spiritual forces which hold sway creatively behind Nature. Goethe began to pursue a way of knowledge which then Rudold Steiner led further in his writings and so laid the foundation for exact Spiritual Science. A Goethean manner of thinking and looking at the world is therefore so fruitful for the therapist.

For Ita Wegman, illness was not a misfortune but a grace, by means of which a transformation, a new development, becomes possible. The higher members of one's being create corrective experiences in the unconscious. But in this time

Im Anbruch des Wirkens für eine Erweiterung der Heilkunst, Natura Verlag, Arlesheim

which is given to him, the higher consciousness also of the sick person should absorb new ideas from the most varied spheres, so long as he is free for a time from service to the world—which means from our normal working life. Besides reading, 'artistic therapy' here plays a significant role. If the therapist is equal to his task, it provides opportunity for a great deal of stimulation. He can with all simplicity and discretion unfold new things to the patient's soul, not in order to instruct him, but in a way similar to that in which Nature herself works, and offer a mode of viewing things which leaves the person completely free.

This may also seem self-evident, but many a person today is so quickly satisfied. If one understands a little of something one believes oneself to be already sufficiently well-grounded, especially in the artistic sphere. But one will very soon become aware that both oneself and the patients lose interest in the repetition of the same thing. The therapeutic capacities and qualities which have been described need by no means to be fully developed, as they certainly grow in the course of one's vocation, but they should not be totally lacking. Much in artistic therapy will be mediated without words through the character of the therapist and the unconscious imitation by the sick person. We are not so cut off from the environment as we believe. From pedagogy we know that the next higher member of the teacher's being always acts on the next lower member of the child's being. Naturally this is valid in a greater measure in youth. The teacher's ego acts, for example, on the astral body of the child, and so on. A remnant of this connection however remains, in that the members of the therapist's being act upon those of the patient. During an illness this is experienced the more strongly. One certinly knows how the appearance of the true doctor already helps the patient, if the doctor has developed the qualities which lead to excellence in his profession; or what a disturbing influence a capricious nurse can have on the life forces of the patient.

As little as the doctor is fully prepared when he has passed his state examination, so little is the therapist when he leaves his college; but, to use Christian Morgenstern's words, 'he must know the direction, he must understand the end in view, otherwise he will be unable to find the way.' (*Er muss die Richtung wissen, er muss das Ziel kennen, sonst kann er den Weg nicht finden.*)

Indications for Therapeutic Treatment

In Rudolf Steiner's descriptions of the evolution of the world, it is during the time of the Old Moon, the planetary condition before that of the Earth, in which colour, or the colour-ether, arises, in which angel beings weave light and darkness into each other. The Old Saturn was still dark and brought forth warmth; in the time of the Old Sun, light came into being and, as a further stage of condensing, air. On the Old Moon, light and darkness were woven into colour and, as the shadow of colour, water came into being. Colour and water stand therefore in a world-historical relationship. When it was still possible to experience in pictures the elemental weaving in Nature, the picture formed itself of angels standing to right and left of the rainbow and with small rainbow chalices catching the Heavenly Water, which like dew is endowed with so much direct cosmic strength. The dew comes into being in a very similar way through the wave of colour-ether—I could also say, the 'purpur' wave—which precedes the sunrise.*

Conscious preoccupation with colour as carrier of the soul element is therefore a 'moistening' of our physical nature. Here is the first far-reaching indication for painting. The one-sided intellectual activity of the man of our time dries him out. When Goethe speaks of 'a dried-up sly person' and characterises the scholar in this way, who only desired to know—'much do I know, but to know all is my ambition'—then this is more than just a poetic comparison. And in view of the fact that the law of the thrice-wise Hermes is valid today in exactly the same way as then, and which he has couched in the clear-cut words 'As above, so below', so it is true that this dryness moves downwards from the soul realm through the etheric processes right into the purely physical substance.

But through the colour-life, not only is 'newly-created water' formed, but the water also comes into movement. That means that the person who associates with colours, stimulates his entire glandular system. The astrality, which through the working with colours slips into the etheric, stimulates movement from within. Accordingly the glandular system breathes better. One can also comprehend the whole glandular activity as a kind of 'submerged' breathing. The in-breathing corresponds to the building-up of the secretion in the glands, and the out-breathing corresponds to the excretion. For the higher members of one's being are always connected in a rhythmical breathing manner with the lower; if they

*Dr W. Bühler, *Nordlicht, Blitz und Regenbogen.*

unite too strongly, they will be crippled. Painting therefore stimulates not only the breathing of the soul-life, but indirectly also the metamorphosis of the breathing upwards and downwards; upwards it is the sense-nerve processes; downwards, the mercurial processes in the fluid organism. Our well-being depends very much on their degree of livelines. When they are congested, we become despondent and also enervated, we lose our appetite because the too weak inner breathing creates too little warmth to make possible the proper assimilation of the substances. This points to a further area where therapy is indicated, which extends from the soul aspect right into the physical-etheric. One can in certain circumstances also lose one's appetite for life and become apathetic towards normal stimuli, a symptom which the stress of our times only too often produces, even already with young people. Then one perhaps takes to abnormal stimulants, which only aggravate the whole situation. The upper metamorphosis of the breathing—the breathing in the senses where we are still 'breathers of light' and through the perception process live with interest in the physical world —is then ill. We also in-breathe the sense world, only that is an even finer breathing process taking place on the etheric level. This needs to be newly ensouled. One sees that painting, and above all the association with colours, encompasses in the broadest healing potential all those tendencies to illness which have to do with a disturbance of the breathing life on all levels. This describes in the first place the upper breathing process.

If one comes from the more general symptoms to the more specialised, so must one include all illnesses which have to do with an unlawful seizing of the breathing and circulation activity—so now the middle sphere—by the petrifying and sclerosis-causing head forces. To this group belongs, to begin with, everything from asthma to all kinds of complaints with a tendency to angina, including genuine angina pectoris; further, the arterio-sclerotic processes in the domain of the circulation; and finally, above all, every kind of cramping. The treatment with medicaments is supported by painting through the fact that one learns consciously to grasp the soul-astral forces by means of the ego, and to divert them towards the outer world through the senses and so to release them. The quality of the artistic activity is naturally also important, for one can always work from the middle sphere to both sides; one can, simply through the technique, bring about a drawing-together or a loosening, relaxation or tension; one can work either in the sense of the forming process of the nerves, or of the loosening processes of the metabolism.

To those who especially need painting belong all whose natures are repressed, everyone with blockages in development. Pathological withdrawal from life, irresoluteness, and a swinging to and fro of the soul moods, find a new direction, because through this active working with colours one calls on the ego, the ruler in the soul, and thus in the first instance comes to decision-making; decisions which have no outer consequences but which even so are one's own decisions, that is to say, which colour one chooses, whether something is beautiful or ugly, whether it harmonises or not, and so on. So, that which later strengthens the whole soul-life, is first practised within the artistic sphere. One finds this significant sentence in the *Psychosophie* of Rudolf Steiner: 'There is nothing which is able so completely to fufil the conditions necessary for a healthy soul-life as the surrender to the Beautiful.'—and he also says: 'Therefore is the experience of the Beautiful such an infinitely expansive, warmth-giving satisfaction.'

But above all, rightly-guided painting engenders in the patient a new experience of the surrounding world, a new connection to the beauty of Nature. If earlier, one has passed everything by with indifference, and if thereby Nature also has become silent, so that one takes home with one no joy from a walk in the woods or over the fields—then very soon some of the patients relate to one that already after the first painting session they learn to see anew; that, for example, they have not known at all how a tree grows, what an artistic theme is—which one can either look for and bring to realisation or put together freely—or how a landscape is formed. In short, a new productive relationship is created to the surrounding world, which is all the more important because in general the patient has not the possibility to travel very much. Then from a possible journey he will bring back not only trivialities which are connected with bodily comfort, but will be awakened to an active observation.

In truth, the painting tuition is able to perform an even more profound service for the sick person. If one succeeds—by the inclusion of a more spiritual thinkng through the artistic handling of the moods of Nature, and their metamorphoses through the times of day and seasons of the year, or of the Elements—in building up in the soul of the sick person the conviction that a deeper meaning, a Divine ordering, holds sway behind the phenomena, then one has created a foundation again for many of the doubting and despairing, empty souls of today on which they are able to stand, through which they can find themselves again, and that is the most important thing. Present-day medicine has no time to foster a comprehending, loving building-up of the soul forces. It is by its very nature, wholly focussed upon diagnostic analysis—in psychology this is also the case. Artistic therapy has however a totally different task. In the etheric body, it should stimulate enlivened breathing in the fluid organisation: a uniting of details into a whole, a 'breathing' drawing-together and loosening; and further,in the astral body, the creation of harmony through the strengthening of the ego in the soul. For all this can only be attained through the ego, which in the artistic process is called upon as the real performer. This ego is spirit, it is the most individual part of us, gentle or strong, egoistic or prepared for sacrifice. The ego is active only in a warmth process; warmth is the only element in which it is able to be present. Joy and enthusiasm allow it to be present, and again form warmth processes which reach as far as genuine physical warmth. Through this, the ego itself gains more ground in the soul. The ego is the drop of Divine creative spirit in us, which is able to maintain itself within itself. This fact plays a great role with the so-called chronic illnesses. They would be much more open to being influenced if it were possible—through the ego—to liberate the astral body from perpetually staring at the malady, and to teach the person so to live with his illness that the ego-consciousness remains as much as possible free from it, and the soul is then able to be filled with other impressions. If an artistic study arises from artistic therapy, so much the better. One should of course never expect quick results, although they are also possible. In general, artistic therapy is a direction-indicator, and then the path will have to be trodden further by the patient himself. The therapist accompanies the sick person for part of the way, but then the latter should of course himself go further. This indicates that artistic therapy is not to be comprehended as though it were concerned with 'a little bit of painting'. The instruction should be built up in a well-considered manner, so that a path becomes recognisable which can lead further. Otherwise the interest very quickly flags.

A further area for therapeutic treatment is indicated by another illness of our time, and this is sleeplessness, especially if it is connected with a complete estrangement of the astral body from the cosmic world, and if during the whole day, only materialistic-mechanistic concepts about the universe live in it. Should it then detach itself in sleep and plunge into the cosmic world, it quickly returns to its former connection with the physical body because of this loss of relationship. But painting has a special relationship to the world of sleep. At night, the astral body expands in the direction of the spiritual behind Nature, which is the lowest cosmic sphere, the Moon-sphere, the first to which we ascend when we leave the body. It is at the same time the etheric world, which forms the bridge to the higher spheres. In this live the colour and form beings in ever-changing Imaginations. The moon mirrors downwards to us, into the Moon-sphere, the whole realm of the sun in pictures. The moon of course belongs to the earth. Her sphere is the intermediate realm which the deceased person also enters when he experiences the looking-back over his life in pictures. Then follows Kamaloka—the living backwards through the times of sleep of our earthly life, in which we have already practised each night, as though in anticipation, the passing of a moral judgement upon the day's experiences. This world, which projects also into our dreams, is the source of experience for painting. We conjure the night into the day in pictures, as Rudolf Steiner once expressed it. Even in earthly life, the nights of the full moon are loosening—nights in which the soul is easily lifted out; this can in certain circumstances lead as far as sleepwalking. But if we grasp the experiences in the etheric world with an awake ego, and form artistically what weaves as the spiritual behind the apearances of our physical earthly world, then we are painters of the future. One should see in this light all Rudolf Steiner's Nature sketches, and then the sense and task of the new art reveals itself, which should make the invisible—that is, the creative forces behind the created world—visible. This means, to continue Nature in creative art.

Within our earthly surroundings, it is especially the being of the plant that helps us on our way. The forces which lead from the plants towards the cosmos with a slight spiralling tendency, as Rudolf Steiner describes it, at night take the human soul with them. How grateful we should be to the plants! If we lovingly paint and study their heavenly forms and cosmic harmonies, then we create in our astral bodies the relationship to the cosmos which we need in order to obtain new forces for the fatigued physical-etheric body which remains lying in bed. These are events on the further side of space and time, and can in the shortest sleep lead us to the boundary of the planetary system. It is a soul-warming thought that roses, lilies, violets and all flowers blossom around us not only for the joy of our senses, but at night for a heavenly ladder on which we are able to ascend. The spiritual world is not at all prosaic, for Nature is the greatest artist and where she works creatively, it is out of profound artistic forces. In the highest spiritual world are the archetypes of the Creation, and here the Creative Word holds sway, as John expresses it. The Creative Word descends through four stages to earthly appearance. From a certain point of view one can say: the Word becomes music, then picture, then spatial appearance in the physical world. This is the metamorphosis of the Creation, which sounds forth also in St John's Gospel. It is the path of incarnation of each spirit, and therefore also of each human ego. It leads from the Saturn-sphere to the Sun-sphere, then to the Moon-sphere and finally to the Earth.

This is all mentioned here because artistic therapy needs a background extending into the spiritual, in order to support the modest activity in the foreground, so that it remains effective and living even if one has ever and again to use the simplest exercises with sick people. Artistic therapy is—and just here I would like this to be remembered—the 'sacrificed art'. This relates to the therapist himself, who is able to nourish the source of his artistic strength and fantasy not on the joy from his own artistic achievement, but from the knowledge of the spiritual connections between illness and destiny, between the macrocosmic forces and their reflections in microcosmic man. Out of veneration for the Fall of Man and the healing of this through Christ—from such thoughts and feelings he draws ever new impulses for this vocation, and nourishes the souls of sick people.

If in the first place in this chapter, the main groups of situations are described where treatment with therapeutic painting is indicated, one should also bear in mind that there is, of course, still a whole range of additional single areas where treatment can also be used. One will however discover by closer observation that in the long run, in the case of all disturbances, one of the previously described processes is in the first place disturbed. By and large, it is the overlapping disturbed processes—i.e., many illnesses interacting—of the working together of the members of one's being which must be treated, not the clinical diagnoses directly. These are too narrowly conceived to be able to give sufficient stimulation to the therapeutic fantasy, for this must in each separate case proceed from the actual situation of the sick person and his spirit-soul disposition.

Therapy for the Illnesses of Our Time

One of the most feared illnesses of our time is cancer and related tumour illnesses. It is not my task to speak about this vast field from the medical point of view. If one observes the tumour-forming process from the viewpoint of the fuctional threefoldness of the human organism, then it appears as an 'overwhelming' by the nerve-senses processes. These turn inwards, an involution process comes into existence, and the result is, in Rudolf Steiner's words: 'The formation of a sense organ in the wrong place', that is, in the metabolic region. When a sense organ is finally developed, the higher members of one's being—ego, astral body and part of the etheric body—loosen themselves from it and, from then on, serve the activity of perception, which is soul process. However, if that should happen in the metabolic region, where the organs must always be wholly penetrated by the higher members and directed from within in their growth, then, instead of a truly human formation, there arises a wild growth of chaotic tissue, indeed, 'suffocated' tissue, because neither does the rhythmic system permeate this place rightly, nor do the astral body and ego organisation regulate the growth.

Dr Werner Kaelin has illustrated this process in his paper published in 1930: *The Prophylactic Therapy for the Cancer Illness* with the following drawing:

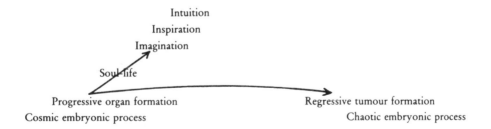

The etheric or life body first builds up the physical body. When this process is finished, the etheric body loosens itself from certain parts, especially from the senses-nerves system and the bones, and henceforth serves the soul life. At first one grows physically, but then a spirit-soul growth begins which lasts until the end of life and allows us to become wise. The loftiest fruit of soul growth today is the development of the higher senses, whose spiritual stages of perception Rudolf Steiner has characterised as Imagination, Inspiration and Intuition—the three stages of higher perception in the spiritual world.

The left arrow in the sketch indicates this direction, in which a regular stream of growth leads upwards from the physical to the soul and spiritual world. This process is disturbed through tumour formation. Instead of leading the forces outwards towards higher evolution, the stream of formative forces turns inwards and an involution process begins. This happens in the precancerous state, and is generally accompanied by depression, and by an increasing anxious awareness of diminishing forces and faculties. People become vulnerable and shy, withdraw, and feel themselves excluded. The inward-turned soul force divines in a dull way the secrets of the blood. In social life, this often leads to inhibited relationships, and to peculiar feelings of guilt—in short, to a deep feeling that the instrument of the soul is out of tune. No longer does the soul rest 'in the peace of God's hand', that is, in spiritual security, but a restless tugging at the fetters of the body ascends as fear from the depths.

Naturally, not all of these symptoms become apparent, they can be hidden or veiled in many ways; but there are hardly any patients who do not have feelings of fear and loneliness and who recognise a decline in their faculties.

Now because each artistic activity calls the ego to the scene and turns the soul outwards, each practice of artistic therapy is therefore of benefit. But painting here plays a still more especial role. The world of colour is indeed the direct expression of the soul world, which the colours reveal—that is, they bring the inwardness of the astral body to outer manifestation. In order to be healthy, the world of 'impressions' must in some way be balanced with the soul's capacity for expresssion. Here the words of Goethe are applicable from his drama *Torquato Tasso*, where he lets the poet burst out with these words:

> *Und wenn der Mensch in seiner Qual verstummt,*
> *gab mir ein Gott zu sagen, was ich leide!*
> (And when Man in his agony becomes speechless,
> A god granted me the possibility of expressing what I suffer!)

The human personality, the ego, the ruler of the soul, is placed between polarities, between the forces of antipathy which bring about distance but also knowledge, and consequently mediate the impressions, and the forces of sympathy which, in the warmth of the will, stream outwards from within. These forces of sympathy need to be stimulated when an involution illness is present. Therefore one chooses colour because it builds the bridge from outside inwards, and from within outwards. It hovers between the heavenly and earthly worlds, between light and darkness, between the inner and the outer. Immersed in colour, one is in the subjective but at the same time also in something objective. It belongs to us and to the world as does the breath, which we take in and again release.

Now one should copy the breathing process in this way even into the technique, and bring action and contemplation into balance. This occurs expeically in the veiling technique, as we have seen. In this method, the picture is woven out of a breathing alternation between a will decision and the observation of the result. This process passes each time over a feeling. The feelings orginating in

34

sympathy have, as bodily reciprocal process, glandular activity. They 'moisten' the physical body to some extent, thereby loosening the hardening processes. Such feelings always set in when the patient gains joy in activity, and when through this he is made warm. Painting creates then a mild fever and therefore acompanies directly the mistletoe therapy, which pursues the same goal from the bodily side—that is to say, it creates a mantle of warmth around the tumour. Painting therapy, rightly guided, provides the same process on the soul level. This of course only becomes effective if it can be carried out over a longer period of time, indeed, when painting becomes a life companion. An inexhaustible source of 'self-knowledge through world knowledge' dwells in this artistic activity, which is able to combine in a slow, continuous process of transformation the tendency of the soul toward involution.

It has ever and again proved helpful to lead sick people to objective Nature pictures—times of day, seasons of the year and similar themes; for example, the plant in its stages of growth, trees as individualities, or to suggest as a theme the variations in the earth's countenance from the pole to the equator. These tasks enable the fantasy to be occupied over a longer period of time with definite connections. In other cases, one prefers to begin with moods of blue, in which the soul feels itself at home and supported. The therapeutic fantasy must in some serious cases find a way, so to speak, from the Moon to the Sun, from the ruler of the night to the shining day-Star. From this picture, the therapeutic endeavour can be grasped.

Then after some time, the souls which are closed up and withdrawn from life express themselves better in that they can now again see Nature rightly, whose beauty they previously passed carelessly by. One can remind them of the lovely words of Caspar David Friedrich:

> In the evening I walk over field and meadow, the blue sky above me and, all around me, green crops and green trees, and I am not alone; for He who created heaven and earth is all around me and His love supports me. (1822 to his wife Karoline).

He has not, generally speaking, painted human beings but the countenance of the earth—the earth which is consecrated through the Mystery of Golgotha. And he himself was an inward-looking spirit, and his art was for him a healing life-content in the same way as it was for Van Gogh, until the sick disposition gained the upper hand and for both brought about a tragic collapse.

In working with such sick people, one does well to take heed that the painting technique 'breathes', that activity and observation alternate, and that neither the lively strong-willed tendency, nor the critical judgement, gains the upper hand. But one should take care that the feeling, which is generally depressed, becomes lightened, the soul uplifted and able to find a new relationship to its surroundings. The creative process, as already mentioned, is always connected with the creation of warmth. Painting produces an opening of the senses to the in-flowing of the cosmic-etheric, which is not physically measurable but active in the etheric body as warming and loosening forces. We have wholly lost the capacity of marvelling at the wonder of Nature—who was revered as a goddess and was still perceived imaginatively a few centuries ago by Brunetto Latini. In wonder lives an inner eurythmy A (ah) gesture, and here the same thing happens, namely, a gentle warming.

Now the illnesses in this group are of longer duration, and pass through various stages. With these sick people it is therefore a question of accompanying them over a longer period of time. It is especially good when patients take up painting as an activity in their free time and consistently work further with it. At the beginning of the cancer process—hence in the precancerous condition—the picture often becomes over-formed, with everything concentrated together, and on some occasions plainly shows the illness process. At the end of the drama, when the sick person wishes to release himself from the body, the pictures become softer, more 'floating', and the form element disappears from them, but the colours then also still build the bridge to the Other Land for the departure of the soul from the earth. Just these patients sometimes find it difficult to be able to release themselves, and therefore experience the colour until the end as a great comfort. One certainly has the impression that the illness is completely overcome in the soul, even though it is not possible to heal the body. But because in spiritual-scientific Medicine we do not regard death as an ending, but as a gateway to transformation, development and a further return, such a thought acquires more weight than would otherwise be the case. This perspective into the future gives all artistic therapy an otherwise unsuspected significance, and is able to console not only the patient but also the therapist when there are limitations to our present endeavours.

Another group of illnesses which one finds in increasing measure today, and which may therefore also be regarded as illnesses of our time, are the degenerative nerve illneses. Compared with other organs, the nerve system has only a reduced power of regeneration, because the life-giving etheric body has partly withdrawn in order to serve as the basis for the consciousness processes. Therefore the bood supply is also weaker, and does not penetrate internally but remains rather as a cloak. The nerve system needs a cooler atmosphere. These are all qualities which, with unfavourable conditions—with or without a preceding inflammatory reaction—can lead to decay and degenerative processes. Here above all belong multiple sclerosis, Parkinson's disease, and other rarer variations of the decay of parts of the nerve system. Of course, artistic therapy is not able to regenerate nerve substance; but it is just these patients who are greatly in need of artistic therapy in order, through the stimulation of the etheric forces, to care for the remaining part, and beyond the physical structure, to strengthen the function. When from above downwards the ego grasps the astral body more strongly, and stimulates the life body to fruitful activity, then one is again able to do much for the future. With all these illness situations which extend over a longer period of time, the important question is, how a person lives through these times, rather than whether he will be cured. The technical age, where all practical manipulations become more and more convenient, is just for that reason well suited to choke the living fantasy. People know less and less what to do with their free time. If one is able to make suggestions which contain a therapeutic element specially suited to them, one prevents them from becoming submerged in their illness. An increasing cramping and fettering of the spirit-soul goes along with multiple sclerosis and related illnesses. Therefore one must go far beyond the special task, and bring about a wider soul nourishment. It is above all necessary to generate soul warmth—and especially to teach the value of the warmth element. In some cases, it is just the healthy life of instinct which no longer exists. The patients love that which encourages their illnesss process. The ego, which makes judgements, has lost the rulership over the wish nature of the astral body. An egoism which is more naive is able through this to expand, and builds up around itself an ego-dominated but limited and fixed world.

But with all these descriptions of the soul aspect of an illness, it should be emphatically stated that here only possibilities are spoken of, and are taken from the distinctive features of the character of the illness. For the individual quality of the higher members of a patient's being decides whether a certain symptom develops more or rather less, or perhaps not at all. It lies far from my wish to label such a sick person with this kind of description. Therefore the therapist also has the strict instruction, never to infringe the personality, but to say everything that must be said through the medium of the art. The therapist should employ great attentiveness through silent observation, in order to find the words with which he can reach the soul level of the sick person. He must demand from himself much more than from the patient. A mature, experienced therapist is needed for such sick people, one who is able to suggest a balance in everything; for what these sick people lack is just this balance, which can only be found and experienced in the ego. What is too big to make smaller, what is too small to make larger; to observe how in Nature everything changes at the right time, how each form retains in correct measure its connection with the whole of creation: these should provide indications for the work.

A further greatly increasing phenomenon in our time is the decay of the spine —the illness of the bones. The skeleton is a nerve formation process which has come to an end, in that it drives the deadening process as far as mineralisation— almost to the total driving out of the life body, although a residue of etheric forces remains in the skeleton, in view of the fact that it will be slowly but continuously rebuilt. The spine, which is the grasping point for the ego's forces of uprightness, is in itself an organ related to the ego organisation. One will find the composition and character described in the section of the book *Rhythmical Massage* referring to the study of man. Here however it is a question of harmonising the acting together and the interpenetration of all the members of the human being. Music carries the laws of the ego into the astral body. Music is able to make a beginning, and painting leads these laws further into the etheric body; both tke place in the stream of warmth. At this stage, we are already on the level of function. In order that the physical may be grasped, modelling may finally be used for a while. One remains quite simple, but does not prescribe two therapeutic arts at the same time. This has nothing to do with what the patient may perhaps do as an amateur in these fields—that remains quite separate from it. In each art, the spiritual element, the ego quality, should be stressed. In painting, one would favour veil painting with the picture standing upright, and the bringing our of clear forms from the previously laid on colour mood, as far as the themes of crystals or architecture. The task of indigo, and similar matters, which are described later, also belong here.

Perhaps it becomes ever more evident, what the nature of the finding of tasks in artistic therapy should be, and that they can only be born from the basis of a deepened study of man through spiritual science. The speech of the members of the human being becomes ever clearer, and becomes the guide in a new sphere of therapy, of which we stand only at the beginning. He who desires perfection or flawlessness, must look at himself in his own great imperfection.

To conclude this chapter: that 'time illness' of the previous century, tuberculosis, should be mentioned. One hardly sees it now in general practice, because it is treated in special sanatoria. Therapists who work there will be able to understand, after all that has already been said, that one would work with strong form to counterbalance the tendency to dissolving form—for example, with geometric drawing, or platonic bodies modelled with plasticine and not with wet clay; also the copying of Dürer's woodcuts and similar works. Painting should not be used at the peak of the illness. Painting is above all not to be used in those cases where a danger of haemorrhage exists, and therefore not during the climacteric if repeated haemorrhage occurs. Then the same rules would apply as for the processes of form dissolution.

If however the cavities are calcified, and if the calcification process has gone too far, then painting again comes in question, controlled and observed as to its effect. The tasks would also preferably contain an element of formed objects, as for instance, the illustration of a story, or travel impressions and other possibilities. Here also the individual situation of the patient must be the decisive factor, not simply the diagnosis.

What patients in the sanatoria pursue as occupational therapy is not here touched upon at all, although there are certain connections.

Painting and the Being of the Moon

It has already been explained in the first volume of *Zur Künstlerischen Therapie*, which refers to the two lectures given by Rudolf Steiner on 29 and 30 December 1914, that painting arises when we push the astral body half-a-stage deeper into the etheric body. Then that art arises which contains within itself the laws of our astral body. The pictorial is 'the outward projection of our inner astral nature', which the Old Moon existence has implanted in us. At that time, the astral body became united with the physical-etheric. In these lectures it is said, for example:

> We experience moods inwardly—sorrow or joy, suggestive and distinctive features from whatever Fate brings us. So do we experience what the painter conjures upon the canvas, which is a reflection of our own inner astral being.

Therefore Rudolf Steiner has taken pains, in the description of the Moon existence in *Occult Science*—as he says—to create a pictorial mood. He says further, in the same chapter:

> If human beings immerse themselves in the nature of the Moon condition, then the deeper relationships between form and colour and the nature of *chiaroscuro* will become apparent, and so they will gain inspiration for the creation of pictures.

The therapist should therefore study the arising of the being of the picture on the Old Moon as, just through this, the sliding of the astral body into the etheric body takes place. The degree of penetration is determined through the healthy sunlike rhythm of the breathing which is in conformity with the ego. Let us look more closely at this arising of the being of the picture. Light and darkness already existed, and angel beings carry now light into darkness, now darkness into light, and through this arose colour, the colour ether or chemical ether or sound ether, on whose wings the astral body given by the Spirits of Movement was 'membered' into the etheric body. The first atributes of the soul arise, desire and aversion accompany the etheric life processes, the wish nature will be slowly developed but guided as yet by the Spirits of Form. In the upper human being, the astral body remains more loosely united, it uses the etheric body as a mirror and that dreamlike weaving of pictures arises, which still mirrors quite truly in pictures the processes of the cosmic environment. In the Moon shadows, genuine symbols are created by the angels, the first form of human consciousness. In his upper part, the human being formed himself as a copy of his consciousness processes. The nerves-senses system of the head is such a complete copy. This is at first a structure of light, which is penetrated by the etheric body. This builds it up into its own instrument. Later, the astral body again destroys it, when it creates consciousness. In contrast, all the remaining organs form themselves under the high influence of the Sun. The Sun in the meantime had withdrawn with the finest substances, and formed an opposition to the Moon. So a duality arises in the human germ. That which develops as the weaving of pictures under the influence of the consciousness conditions, lifts itself out as a kind of head. The Moon begins to revolve, so that the human germ is alternately exposed to the Sun, and then again, in turning away from the Sun, is able to come to itself. The Moon human beings themselves also wander around their planet. On the side shone on by the Sun, there is formed everything which does not stand under the influence of consciousness. There, the Moon humanity lives in blissful devotion to the World Harmony. At the end of this Sun period the pictures, which faded during the Sun's influence, become more distinct again, and a kind of awakening to oneself takes place; the angel guiding the consciousness is experienced as a kind of 'Group Ego' and is visible in a picture. These cosmic forces work inwards through the senses and, as already mentioned, develop the foundation of the nerve system. The path from these cosmic dream-pictures to our present-day object consciousness is the path through the closer approach of the astral body, the taking in of the Luciferic influence, being cut off from the cosmos, and the beginning of egoism, with the consequences of error, illness and death.

This disturbing influence happens in the repetition of the Moon period during Earth evolution—that is, in the Lemurian time—which took place on a continent in the region of the Indian Ocean, and which only towards the end of the period acquired firm ground. That which is described in the Paradise myth as the 'expulsion' is a long world process of the slow descent of human souls into physical bodies, who are able to wander over the now mineralised surface of the earth.

All the old Mysteries have known of this process of becoming. Especially the Egyptians remembered this Lemurian time. They knew that all illness came from a corruption of the star-body, which no longer mirrored cosmically the world forces. The healing in the so-called 'Temple Sleep' existed with them. The astral body which was lifted out of the nerve-senses system was, through the Temple ceremonies, led in front of Isis, that is, before the picture of the pure cosmic Star-body as it was before the Fall of Man. Isis is the picture of this cosmic astrality, the pure archetype, the World Soul. On this, the deformed astral body of the patient should and could correct itself. The physical-etheric body was still at that time softer and more impressionable than it is today, and therefore this correction experienced in the Temple Sleep could, on re-awakening, bring about healing on the etheric and physical body.

It will immediately be understood that this was only possible during a certain

40

time. Due to the deeper descent of mankind, it was already in the Greek epoch no longer possible. It is true that in the Mysteries of Asklepios, the Greeks still accompanied the astral body of the sick person in the Sleep, but no longer to the far spaces of the cosmos, to Isis, but only as far as her more humble sister, later known as Natura, the spiritual counterpart of our earthly Nature. At the place where the sick person tarries overnight, his astral body is drawn to its remedy. In falling asleep, when the astral body loosens itself from the sick body, the person dreams about his illness. On awakening, he is able to dream of his remedy—for example, in the picture of a plant. So this Greek period represents the transition from a purely spiritual method of healing to the first use of physical remedies. Through the perception of the dreams, the Greek priest had already experienced the diagnosis through the falling-asleep dream, and through the awakening dream, the therapy. Hippocrates, as he himself says, brings these mysteries to a close. He still knew the Egyptian methods, although they were certainly already decadent at that time.

If one lifts one's gaze to this origin of our picture consciousness, one is able to gather a great deal about the single stages of these events from the fact of the slow coming into being of the earthly, and the hardening of our picture world from the metamorphosing cosmic imges to our limited physical object-consciousness with stable sense-pictures. In addition, one can gather much therefrom about the direction in which, in the future, these pictures must again be enlivened. The purification of the astral body, the healing of the consequences of the Fall of Man, will be mirrored anew in our picture world; this time however, the astral body will be guided not by priests and doctors, but by the individual ego through knowledge, and also through slow transformation by therapeutic exercises.

Here lies a significant future task of artistic therapy (this refers to all the arts). All activities in the Mercury-half of the earth should flow from the ego-consciousness and its corresponding stage of knowledge, and what is more, should receive a certain impulse from Mercury. What we here and now practise as therapeutically-applied art, is time-related and will alter. But the deeper meaning of these activites will not alter; artistic therapy should accompany mankind, as Raphael accompanied the young Tobias. It must reckon with the path of destiny in each individual patient. Should it become only superficial, or even applied with intellectually thought-out fixed tasks for certain diagnoses, then it has not been understood.

The Earth's destiny begins with the repetition of the Moon development in the Lemurian period, when the ego submerges itself into the three sheaths; and after the separation of the Moon from the Earth, souls slowly return again to the Earth. The soul bears the ego downwards. In the soul we experience it inwardly. Polarity comes with the soul; above is the mirroring process, the imaging element; below, the inward movement on the basis of all that which is connected with digestion. In the warm centre of the heart we feel our humanity, the eternal Entelechy, the Measure, which characterises the Master. Everything, including the best, can be too much or too little. The old conception of virtue was 'the middle as the Measure'. Where can one better practise this than in painting? Rudolf Steiner once compared painting to the tightrope dance, for one can continually fall down to one side or the other. But everything in this area is certainly still in the domain of the play of the breathing. Therefore painting as a practised activity brings about a humanising of the soul qualities. Consequently, painting was so categorically included by Rudolf Steiner in pedagogy, so that children lose the inhuman tendencies towards a lack of love on the one side, and to cold abstraction on the other. Today, the kind of painting practised in the Waldorf School is a culture-therapy element of the first importance.

Now because the astral body—as we have already shown—must again destroy its instrument, the nerve-senses system, which it formed in the Moon period, in order to create earthly consciousness, therefore we must ever and again sleep, and draw the astral body out of its instrument in order to regenerate it. But in sleep the astral body plunges into that spiritual world which lies behind the sense world. Rudolf Steiner speaks of this world in a lecture of 12 September 1920 in Dornach:

> This world fires us when we paint. Behind the sense world are not atoms and molecules, but spiritual beings...what emerges in painting is the restoration of the supersensible, a revelation in our spatial environment and, from outside space, the spiritual world penentrating us—the world in which we find ourselves between falling asleep and awakening.

It is also the first world in which we awaken when in death we have stepped across the threshold. One might think that all this lies too far away and is of value only to the free artist; but he who does not know the connection of the artistic to the spiritual world, will also be unable to discover the modification for the individual concrete case in such a way that the task signifies something essential for the sick person. In painting, one should not have fixed exercises, but a therapeutic fantasy. The transitions between art and healing art in the sphere of painting, which stands so near to the operation of the middle region of the human being, are also expecially fluid. Here, therefore, one should proceed in a specially individual manner, since one is not dealing with diagnoses but with human beings and their treatment.

But if I go further to other outer colour treatments through radiation and similar methods, then the effect is quite otherwise. On this, there is already a somewhat detailed literature.

In artistic therapy, and especially in painting, neither the abstract intellectual-scientific, nor the moral-religious, ought to come into the foreground. It should become effective from out of the free artistic centre. Only so does it bring about for the soul a meaningful peace within itself, and a relationship with the world. Through the stimulation of the individual creative activity will the ego, the ruler of the soul forces, be strengthened, and an up-building be brought about, instead of uncertain analysis. What so many people lack is composure, inner peace and certainty. Our time is tearing the soul to pieces, and is creating uncertainty and desolation in the soul. In order to meet these problems, medicine in the future will need to have far greater recourse to artistic therapy, because only with that is it possible to reach the soul and spirit disturbances, through which the physical illnesses—which we have learnt to suppress—will be relieved.

I would like to close this chapter with a brief reference to the deepest impression about the spiritual background of painting, which Rudolf Steiner gave to us in the small pamphlet: *The Nature and Being of the Arts.* This is the rendering of an imaginative experience of a human being who appears as the representative of Art, side by side with a representative of Science.

It is shown in sucession, how this person meets the individual arts at the three higher stages of knowledge. In Imagination, she sees the Being, through Inspiration, she hears It speak to her and entreat her to go forward to Intuition—that is, to union with the Being. Through the latter, she is then able in each case to engender a new capacity in human beings. It is said in this essay:

Another figure came up to her, even stranger and still more remarkable than the preceding one. Quite strange and remarkable. Something streamed out of It which felt like the warmth of love, and again something that produced quite a chilling effect.

In Inspiration, the figure said, among other things:

I am called Intuition, and I come hither from a far realm. And in that I have taken my way from a far realm into the world, I have descended from the realm of the Seraphim.

This figure of Intuition was from the Beings of the Seraphim. And when union with the Being had taken place, the figure said to the woman who experienced all this:

Because thou didst this, thou art now capable of endowing men with that faculty which is painting fantasy. Through this, thou hast become the archetype of the Art of Painting. Through this, thou wilt be able to kindle a faculty in men, to bestow it upon one of their senses, the eye, which contains something in itself which will not be affected by thought activity from the individual human selfhood—something which the comprehensive thinking beyond the material world has in itself—and thou wilt be able to bestow that sense, after thou hast the painting fantasy in thyself. And this sense will be able to perceive, shining through the surface of things which otherwise appear lifeless and soulless, their soul being.

Then follows a description of this faculty in detail—that one so conjures the colour on to the surface that through it, something of the inward nature of the colour speaks, in so far as everything in this sphere moves from within outwards. One can then in tranquility transform soul movement, holding fast everything which is changeable. But the most important thing was stated in these words— that the eye has something in it like a subconscious thought-capacity, which is an etheric activity, and the comprehensive thinking beyond the material world is World thinking, and has not been through the Fall of Man. So a part of the

Paradisal ether, something entirely Sun-like, lives in the eye, not spoiled by our egoism,, something selfless, something innocent and virginal. Through this, and through the fact that the archetype is so exalted that it can be found only in the highest Hierarchy, with the Spirits of Love, the Seraphim, one is able to sense the soul-enobling character of painting, the art which in times past has so devoutly served Religion.

In the first instance, the consideration of painting leads into the Mooon sphere, into our night world, whose soul experiences give inspiration for painting. But the revelation of the archetype leads far higher, right into that world where the First Hierarchy alone was absolute, into the Saturn world—also already recognisable in the characterisation through warmth and frosty cold. Saturn is 'the Father of Colours', who in the World Midnight causes our eternal being to appear in its individual colours. This connection is scenically represented by Rudolf Steiner in his fourth *Mystery Play*. Here the Saturn sphere shines forth in many colours; and each soul which is preparing again for the descent through the planetary spheres, shines forth in the colours of the aura, which reveals his inner qualities.

A healer should ever and again allow the spiritual connections to pass through his soul, in order that the Mercury forces, which are the messengers from the heights to the depths and vice versa, may be livingly preserved in him.

The Individual Colours

The whole realm of colour, but also each individual colour, has two sources, the light and the darkness. Darkness originated in primeval times, it is Saturn-like, cosmic Will pulses through it, it condenses itself in the course of its evolutionary creation towards matter. Finally, matter is the outward appearance of Will; inwardly, matter is Will, as is stated in the lecture of 5 December 1920 in Dornach. That which the Thrones once gave was the Will-like material element, a germinating world, born out of one element which 'using a more oriental expression of the matter could be called Love' (10 December 1920). Cosmic Will is paternal World-Love. Light, on the contrary, is thought-filled Nature, it originated in the Sun epoch, and cosmic thinking, World thinking, lives in it. And when they interweave, colour arises—a revelation of the World soul as cosmic feeling. In feeling, both elements are interwoven. Each feeling has a knowledge aspect and a will aspect. And when the ego lives in feeling, so it creates the harmony between the two poles of human existence, between thinking and doing. While I write this, I have not only Rudolf Steiner's colour lectures in mind, from whose comprehensive contents one is able to create unceasingly, and a detailed study of which belongs to the professional basis of the therapist, but I have also in mind my various conversations with the painter Liane Collot d'Herbois. She was, at the beginning of her artistic career, closely connected with the impulses of Ita Wegman, and worked for years in a curative home in England. She was therefore as a painter very close to therapy. So her art also, in which she especially developed veil painting, has a great culture-therapy quality. Liane Collot d'Herbois gave instruction over many years in our school in Boll, so that much of what now follows stems from this instruction and from many conversations. It was certainly significant for her life work that she was born in Tintagel—that locality where once, in the play of colours in the Elements above the sea, King Arthur's Knights of the Round Table experienced imaginatively the approach of the high Sun Spirit, the Christ, and His penetration of the ether-aura of the earth.

When Liane Collot spoke about colours, everthing was illuminated with spiritual reality, but illustrated from a rich abundance of Nature observations, so that the feeling for colours turned lovingly towards the earth without forgetting the heavens.

The colours of the rainbow will now be considered one after the other, and something from the richness of their possible characteristics, which can meaningfully enliven colour for the pupil, will be brought into relief. Sometimes this begins with Rudolf Steiner's characterisation, which he expressed in the lecture of 1 January 1915 in Dornach, and from which the following quotations are taken.

But in view of the fact that one should always proceed from the totality, something will first be said about the whole colour-bow. In yellow-red, the rainbow has its stimulating, active, raying-out side, and its life then becomes fully portrayed in green, even though green is still the 'dead image of life'. But blue does not ray towards me, but has an 'outstreaming', a 'space-making', quality; it needs boundaries, so that it prefers to be darker at the edges and lighter towards the centre. Life, which is represented by green, paralyses itself and goes back, through a kind of death, to the spirit, to 'purpur' or lilac. There are always paths of the soul which, in passing through the rainbow, play between spirit and matter. As the planetary world circles between the Zodiac and the earth, so is the rainbow—which is membered in a sevenfold way—also a copy of its spheres, on account of which, not only one colour belongs to a planet—it is always a question of from which standpoint, and on which level, they are being described. Each colour contains once again the whole rainbow, so that not seven, but fortynine, colour tones result. Each colour can have a blueish or reddish nuance, but it is much better in the first instance to imagine this fact only as a fleeting manifestation, rather than to contruct schemes with the intellect and, so to speak, to play with coloured pearls. For as with music, the reality lies between the tones, so is this the case with the transitions between the colours. This does not contradict the fact that identification with one colour gives a special tendency to the soullife. These tendencies one is able to use therapeutically.

Now to begin with Rudolf Steiner's words:

> If one identifies oneself with blue, one would go through the world with the desire, as one proceeded, to overcome the egoism in oneself, to become macrocosmic. One would feel happy to remain in this condition to meet the Divine Mercy. Thus one would go through the world feeling as if blessed with the Divine Mercy.

Blue is 'the lustre of the soul' and is able to expand in the soul in its entirety, to widen out of the constraint of the earthly, becoming even more macrocosmic. Calmness proceeds from experience of blue, because it is the colour of the knowledge side of our soul capacities. The restless soul is able to collect itself together for self-assessment. Blue has many stages between heaven and earth. Cobalt blue is the most heavenly, then the 'Fra-Angelico-Blue', which at a certain time replaced the gold background—the sunlight weighted down to gold—so that the picture, for the observer, was no longer experienced imaginatively in light outside his own self, but turned inwards into the soul—a process of deeper intensification. Cobalt blue therefore in the world of plants is a volatile colour, and the blossoms wither quickly.

All the other nuances of blue lie between cobalt blue and indigo, and that is an extensive world. Blue can be either warm or cold, Prussian blue being the coldest; it presses toward form—indeed, it can become very physical in its effect to the point of denser, coarser materiality. One sees from this that it does not suffice only to say: one should paint blue—it is more important 'how' one paints it. In our natural-scientifically orientated time, we all incline towards blue; it is receptive—the mantle for our conscious soul contents. That is to say, blue represents the entire soul forces of the upper astral body, in so far as we knowingly shape them in ourselves. On the one side, blue inclines—as do the head forces—towards concentration and towards the earth element. The earth as a whole passes as a 'blue star' through the world of space. Seen from outside, her dark nucleus gleams blue through the illuminated gloom of her covering of air. The space travellers have brought us impressive pictures of this. On the other side, blue expands into indefiniteness. It draws us full of longing into the distance, hence the longing for the spiritual homeland resides in the depths of each soul so long as it remains in earthly incarnation, only it is covered over by the variety of nearer-lying things. This leads back to Rudolf Steiner's characterisation that we become more macrocosmic through identification with blue.

In view of the fact that these descriptions can only betoken a stimulation, without in the least pretending to be complete, so we will pass on to the next colour: green.

First of all, Rudolf Steiner's words (Christiania, 18 and 20 May 1923: 'Colours as the Revelation of the Psychic in the World'):

> Now let us look at green, in which we have, so to speak, a kind of cosmic word, proclaiming how life weaves and has its being in plants. In observing how life works its way through dead particles to create thereby the plant image, we recognise green as the dead image of life.

And in addition, 1 January 1915, at Dornach:

> If one identifies oneself with green, and goes with green through the universe, which can quite easily be done by gazing at a green meadow and trying to shut out all else and concentrate entirely upon the green meadow, and then by trying to dive down into the green meadow—observing the green as if it were the surface of a coloured sea and then diving down into the green—when one tries to live in this way in the world, one experiences an inner strengthening of that which one is, in that particular incarnation. One experiences an inner increase of egoism, an inner stimulation of the power of egoism.

One only needs to allow these sentences of Rudolf Steiner, with their repetitions, to act upon one, and one will be led to the activity of the etheric body, the life body, which we draw towards us for each separate incarnation shortly before conception.

The colour green, which mirrors the earthly life of the plants, has something calming within it—one feels ground under one's feet. In Goethe's colour circle, blue and yellow condense downwards to green, towards the earth. Through this, a stable equilibrium is also created. Only when one became able, through the ego, to rule, order, and make inward one's own soul-life, could one see green outwardly. The conquest of the soul-life by means of the ego, a work which lasts through the whole post-Atlantean culture period, will be accompanied by a mastery of the outer seeing of colours. Until the time of Greece, all colours have a reddish tinge, because the etheric body is still active in the senses, and dream-like clairvoyance is mixed with perception. With the advent of the ego in the intellectual soul in Greek times, not only does the glance towards the outer world become clear, but also the soul-survey clarifies towards the birth of philosophy. But there is at the same time a kind of 'standstill' which was painfully experienced; the feeling of being caught in the earthly sphere begins with green. But in this green a new life is able to begin, and therefore Rudolf Steiner could also say that green belongs to the Christ colours, to the image colours black, white, peach-blossom and green, which have all become silent and plunged into the realm of death. But from the very same foundation, new life is able to rise in green; 'Resurrection green' is a green with a kind of turquoise and emerald nuance, as it was painted by the Master of the Isenheim Altar. Death, but also redemption, is the secret of green.

There is therefore in green a kind of timeless peace and stability; when it grows too rigid, it leads to the 'green table' of abstract judgements and theories, which without examination withdraw themselves from reality.

In therapy, green brings about an enlivening of the senses-organisation, a calming of the soul, a certain seclusion and a finding of ground under one's feet. Eye patients show especially good results with green where the organ itself has need of an enlivening and inner strengthening, so that the astral body and ego are better able to seize it in the act of seeing. The pure emerald green does not exist in the plant world, but can be found among reptiles and insects, where the astral body determines the form and colour. With the sensible/moral after-effect of a colour, which is connected with the formation of complementary colours, naturally the quality of a colour is decisive, so that the plain intellectual statement that green produces peach-blossom refers always to a saturated middle tone. Yellow-'May-green', and the blue-green of certain fir trees, have very different results, because the light element has been drawn into the darkness in very different degrees. The Romans, so it is said, loved the dark green; they stand at the deepest point of incarnation right into the metabolism, which supports the earth-will and also draws the limbs more strongly into the earth's field of action. Marching, they conquered their Roman empire.

While with green we are entirely on the earth, with yellow we ascend into the light. Yellow is the first gentle darkening of the light. Again, Rudolf Steiner's words:

> If it is a yellow surface and we immerse ourselves in it and go through the world as a yellow-filled person, then we feel in this experience of yellow as if —so I would like to describe it—we were transferred to the beginning of our time-cycle. We feel: now you are living with the forces out of which you have been created, when you entered upon your first earth incarnation. One feels an affinity between what one was during the whole of the earth's existence and what comes towards one from the world into which one carries the yellow oneself.

The eternal core of the human being glimmers through these words, the ego aware of itself, the spirit of man. Pure yellow is therefore noble and joyful, it turns towards the world in order to give something to it, and also to acquire something. Yellow shines into the darkness, into death. It is the 'lustre of the spirit' and brings its semblance into the picture. Paul Klee has said: 'yellow is an endless gaining of ground'; this is also a quality of the human spirit which seeks its own development. Yellow has something strongly uniting, a Mercurial quality—if one may put it so. In China, it is the colour of the highest honour. But all this applies only in the span of pure yellow to yellow with a reddish tinge. Should yellow have only the slightest tendency towards green and become dirty, then it falls from its throne into degradation and becomes the colour of bankrupts, prostitutes and other ostracised people (the Star of David). In painting, yellow on its own is not easily managed, it will have no boundaries but wishes to radiate from a concentrated middle-point. So other colours must set the boundaries, but it will nevertheless still shine over them where veil painting is concerned. Then its uniting nature comes so rightly to expression.

In therapeutic painting, one always takes care that in the course of the work yellow does not lose its uniting strength and its joyous inclination to give, so remaining pure. As the spirit desires to move in freedom, so yellow also does not want to become squeezed in; but it is also able to lose itself in complete surrender to the other colours. If yellow becomes weighed down to gold, condensed, it repesents the Sun-forces of the ego-sphere on the physical plane. The other colours stand out from the gold background of the early Middle Ages, not very strongly connected together but placed in the space as single individualities, before there was perspective. The blue backgrounds of Giotto and other Masters such as Fra Angelico drew the picture, as already stated, more into the interior of the soul.

If yellow is enhanced to orange, if it warms itself slightly by means of one of the spirit-bearing warm souls, then we feel something which Rudolf Steiner has characterised in the following words:

> If we sink ourselves into an orange surface and become one with it, we shall not have the feeling of Divine Wrath bearing down upon us (as with red), but we shall have the feeling that what meets us here, though having something of the seriousness of wrath in a modified form, is yet desirous of imparting something to us, instead of merely punishing us—of furnishing us with inner strength. If we go out into the universe and become one with orange, we move in such a way that with every step we take, we feel: through this sensation, through this living in the forces of orange, we experience ourselves in the world in such a way that we become stronger and stronger, not merely that the Divine Judgement is shattering us. So that what comes towards us from orange brings not merely punishment but a strengthening quality. In this way we live with orange in the universe. Then we learn to apprehend the love of life, the inner aspect of things, and to unite these with ourselves. Through living in red, we learn to pray; through living in orange, we learn understanding, the longing for knowledge of the inner nature of things.

This description by Rudolf Steiner shows especially clearly that it has nothing to do with an intellectual learning of the facts. That could be dealt with in three lines. It is concerned with how one can reach, through the experience of the colour, an effect on the etheric body, on the life-sphere. With the forces of the middle-sphere, the Druid priests once investigated, in the shadow of the dolmen—in order to eliminate the physical light—the spiritual in the sunlight. The domain of feeling must be refined from its exclusively subjective character to become again an instrument of knowledge. Feeling comprehends in a rhythmical manner, in a time process, for which the modern intellectual person does not allow time. He cannot wait. To be able to wait is the great strength of the ego. All haste comes from the astral body, which is unable to say 'no'. Whoever really works with these colour exercies, implants his spirit more deeply into his soul, thereby creating a harmonious soul-mood and thus also, a healthier one.

After everything that has been said about orange, one will understand that it plays an important role in therapeutic painting, because yellow is very often initially warmed by it. In the same way that each day we take the glow of the evening sun with us into the night, so should the sick person experience more frequently the stronger, warmer colours, without in any way exaggerating these indications. Orange in large surfaces is not pleasant; but one can decorate passages and stairwys with orange wall colours, because there one is in movement, one passes through. There is also a gentle impulse to movement in orange, but without it causing emotion. In the delicate blue of the etheric complementary colour, the mood of the longing for knowledge is portrayed, which we awaken. Orange is in any case a mood which is outward-turning. In the evening sky, we receive with the orange tones the last warm greeting of the departing sun—a poignant experience. In the Alpine glow, this is enhanced to 'purpur'. At the time when it was still possible to see imaginatively the elemental beings and the beings of the Third Hierarchy, who rule in this glow, the legends of the 'Rosengärten' arose out of this phenomenon——the roses blooming mysteriously on this peak—as well as 'König Laurins Reich' and also the 'Triglav Rosen'. The Triglav is a mountain in the southern chain of the Alps, which today is in Jugoslavia. The legend of its roses, and the ibex with the golden horns which guards the garden of the fairies, inspired Baumgarten to write the poem 'Zlatorog', to which Rudolf Steiner has often drawn attention. In the lonely Alpine valleys, as also with the Celts, a certain clairvoyance for the Nature beings was preserved longer than with the rest of mankind; and so there are countless Alpine legends connected with definite places and phenomena, which originate from the experience of the activity of different elemental beings. Naturally, these also slowly became intellectualised and lost their genuine quality. It is interesting how differently the morning Aurora affected men's consciousness. The evening glow is a departing greeting, the Aurora something prophetic, a call of destiny: What will the day bring? Because today feeling has become suppressed rather than refined, so the modern intellect smiles about these impulses from the deeper layers of the soul; but they contain more truth than is attainable by us in our uppermost level through purely natural-scientific thinking on the basis of pure perception. The latter, on the other hand, investigates the physical plane in a way that no clairvoyance is able to do. The one must be widened through the other to a spiritual-scientific observation of the world, which had in Goethe so eminent a representative that Rudolf Steiner could form a direct connection with him.

Let us return to the intensification of orange to red. The intensification of the inner emotion, the striving outwards, since it corresponds to the will side of the soul-life, leads to vermilion, which acts in a heavy, earth-bound, iron-related, emotional and passionate manner, as far as aggressiveness. The more we move over from vermilion to carmine, the nearer we approach to 'purpur'. Once again, the experience of red as given by Rudolf Steiner:

> Let us simply take the case when we direct our gaze to a gleaming surface evenly covered with strong vermilion red. Let us assume that we succeed in forgetting everything else round us and concentrate entirely on the experience of this colour, so that we have the colour in front of us not merely as something that works upon us, but as something wherein we ourselves are, with which we ourselves are one...
>
> If we float through the world as red, and have become indentical with red, if one's own soul and also the world is entirely red, we shall not be able to help feeling that this red world in which one is oneself red, is pierced with the substance of Divine Wrath, which pours upon us from every direction on account of all the possibilities of evil and sin in us. We shall be able to feel we are in the illimitable red spaces as in a judgement court of God.

And then when the reaction comes, and the experience passes over into a moral experience, so it can only be that one would like to characterise it with these words: one learns to pray. Then Rudolf Steiner leads the experience further to the perception of a being full of goodness and mercy, who appears in the centre of the dispersing red in a kind of pink-violet, this streaming outwards from the centre and shading-off—if one wishes to represent the experience pictorially in colours.

Especially important with red is the fact that it is able to uplift and ennoble itself through all degrees from the earthly and dense vermilion through scarlet and carmine to deep rose red, and finally to 'purpur'. There is much darkness in red, much will and an enduring warmth. Our soul answers spontaneously when, in the earthly green of our environment, red appears, be it only a red sunshade or a grazing cow; for the green remains under our feet, but the red appears upon it as a living dynamic being, something congenial. Only when too strong, it works in a threatening manner and attacks us.

Physiologically, the observation of a saturated red surface allows the forces of the metabolism to rise up towards the head; this becomes rather more permeated with blood, and consequently the nervous system is attacked. The astral body seizes the etheric body in the circulation of the fluids rather more strongly, and the blood spreads out to the periphery as far as the skin and the senses. This is accompanied by a sense of cheerful well-being when it happens in moderation; if the process becomes blocked or dammed up, then anger arises, a lively assertion of the ego. Red is 'the lustre of life', as it is described in Rudolf Steiner's colour theory, and moreover, of the earthly life. Earthly life is a plunging into darkness; light suffers red. Goethe speaks of the deeds and sufferings of light, and from this one can feel how red contains cosmic pain or wrath, while blue in this connection signifies a deed, it illuminates the darkness and lightens it to blue. The paths of our soul pass over red in the darkness, over blue again to the light, ascending and descending, for red and blue blood are equally necessary. In the red oxygen-rich blood, the astral body plunges into the denser etheric body; in the blue blood, rich in carbon dioxide, it partly frees itself again;—the head is the 'most blue', one might say, the spleen and kidneys entirely red,—the heart, on the other hand, restores the balance and therefore gives to the regulating ego a freedom space. If one allows this to reveal itself in colour, one would experience peach-blossom, the diluted 'purpur'. Here sympathy and antipathy are silent because the ego holds sway over it. Peach-blossom, the rose-red, can mount gradually from the palest briar-rose tone to the darkest rose colour in the darkness. Yes, we can rightly speak of a 'purpur' darkness. The Spirit, which was at the beginning of the world, was spiritual-physical. It contained the laws of matter as well as those of the spirit. It was active in the Saturn-fire of the Thrones. The 'purpur' darkness is warm, imbued with spirit. Rembrandt was acquainted with it. He understood many secrets of light and darkness which are only given to the pupil of the Spirit. From this, one may draw the conclusion that he met a Master, as with all great heralds of the future, whether it be through the word or through art or another medium.

Throughout the whole of her painting, the artist Collot d'Herbois was attracted to 'purpur', magenta, as being a question concerning the revelation of a threshold of consciousness between a sensible and a supersensible world. There are observations by Rudolf Steiner which imply that the person who sees peach-blossom—in this case as flesh-colour—already experiences something supersensible. For the spirit in man brings about this colour; and one errs profoundly if one thinks that a simple pink, perhaps that of a piglet, can possibly be compared with the human flesh-colour. Magenta reveals itself quite differently in the plant kingdom and in the mineral kingdom as the manifestation of something spiritual, through the rose on the one hand, and through the tourmaline or rose-quartz on the other. In former times only priests and kings were allowed to wear 'purpur'. Phoenicia is considered to be the first country where, in olden times, 'purpur' was produced from snails and material dyed with this—the land of the Phoenix Mysteries where one understood death and resurrection in the passing of the human ego through its earthly destiny. Near to 'purpur', but heavier and more serious, inwards-turning, violet finally appears as the manifestation of the darkness. In its depths, the soul finds in devoutness, surrender to the Divine Will. One's own aggressive willing becomes quiet. Liane Collot d'Herbois used to say:

> The violet quietness can slowly concentrate, and substance arises. With this, one is in the darkness of the will-sphere. There we draw forth the courage for the earthly goals of all religions, if one identifies oneself in deepest seriousness

with violet, and then again comes to the light, ascending, so to speak, from the violet.

Violet acts powerfully on the will. Experience has shown that psychically ill people can lose themselves in violet, and in painting, can remain stuck fast in it. In curative painting, it would be used only very occasionally, for in most cases one has to lead the sick person out of this colour if he has been overwhelmed, psychically and physically, by the hardening forces which are reflected in deep violet. With pale lilac, the exact opposite shows itself; it floats directly upwards, and shows its relationship to blueish-peach-blossom. Modern man has no special connection either to the one side or the other; and therefore in the psychological test by Heinrich Frieling it is considered also to be a 'disturbing colour' because it leads towards the psychic boundary situations, in the darkness of matter or in the etheric levity.

The violet stone, the amethyst, is a helper against ego weakness, and this becomes manifest especially through mania—the unruly astral body. One could in addition mention that the deep violet of the Church vestments, as insignia for the Offering and Atonement, stands for the unconditional surrender of one's own will to the will of God.

One would like to say at this point that brown should be appreciated. The complementary colour to the violet is a delicate yellow, which becomes brown if one mixes it with red and blue. It is the deepening of both sides of the spectrum, not to a living green but to earth brown. Brown is a warm colour, almost akin to gold—which is also a condensing from yellow, the lustre of the spirit. Brown represents the 'good earth', the upholding and enduring earth, the 'all-digesting' earth. In therapy, one can also use brown for everyone who has lost the ground from under his feet. But never will one colour of the therapeutic selection be used singly, but employed to build up a picture, so that a conversation can take place. Brown is also the colour of the penitent's robe, he who bears his sins with resignation and goodwill. It is true that brown is not a colour of the rainbow, but one can allow it to arise through mixing, in which the earthy vermilion plays a special role. The warm brown teaches us to love the earth. Brown is the colour of wood, which the plant world gives to us as the substance of the upright gesture, the cosmic prototype for the posture of our ego. The first pillars were papyrus plants bundled together, and this fact also brings brown nearer to green.

There is yet another colour which reveals a secret of the darkness, and that is indigo; it lies between dark blue and violet. In our gradual conquest of the seeing of the outer colours, indigo is the last stage; and the corresponding soul quality which we have finally acquired in connection with the bodily functions, is the so-called 'pure perception'. At the beginning of our fifth culture period, which serves the development of the consciousness soul—to be achieved by the ego at the boundary of the physical body—the last remnants of the imaginative forces disappeared from the perception of the outer world. We are able to see the physical world 'naked', as is necessary, and is a basic condition, for the beginning of natural science. With this, the ego stands solitary over against the physical world, at the boundary of the sub-sensible world where the real perceptions cease and only the calculable obtains—where therefore theories begin, because there in no more 'appearance'. But at this boundary the ego can discover itself in full awakeness and independence. Now indigo has an especial relationship to the sense process, to the world of Saturn, to the mineral-physical plane, to the ending of the creation of this Saturn world, of these World Creative Father forces. Clouds, bones and ashes are indigo-coloured, and also distant mountains when the air is especially humid. With indigo, this blackish-blue, there comes already a death presentiment in the soul; black would be the full spiritual image of death, as one of the four image colours—black, white, peach-blossom and green. But the blue tone in indigo allows this colour to appear as a soul experience. When we observe indigo clouds, we suspect something threatening behind them, and that stamps indigo as the boundary colour to an invisible world of forces—in Nature, the forces of Pluto. Lava is also indigo-coloured. One experiences the spiritual content of indigo best when one paints with it oneself. The first great painter to use indigo was El Greco. It was hazardous, because for him, behind the indigo there was even the threat of the Inquisition. For the Church declared this colour 'the devil's colour'. This is also a truth in so far as Ahriman is the justified Lord of Death, and one enters his kingdom when one recognises oneself as an individual ego on the physical plane. From the fifteenth century there began the conquest of the earth with its materials, and their mastery through the machine culture. At the same time we began to see indigo outwardly. Children do not see it at all until about the twelfth year, when for the first time the higher members grasp so deeply in, that pure perception can arise in the senses, which alone is able to nourish and build up a scientific consciousness. We thereby investigate, in our technical age, the naked realities of the material world and control them through technical science. Parts of a landscape which earlier was ensouled, die into barren factory terrain. The picture of the world changes. Cities are built, somewhat like heads with an accumulation of intelligence and teaching centres. This all belongs in the world of indigo. Man must go through the natural-scientific consciousness, through the contact with the threatening forces of the inside of the earth, in the centre of substance. All this, gathered together into a sensible/supersensible feeling, allows itself expression in indigo. And because indigo is one of the colours of the rainbow, it has the possibliity of artistically ensouling this whole world, of artistically lifting it up, yes, of trans-figuring it. In the chapter on the Teaching Plan (Lehrplan), there is an exercise with indigo which illustrates what is here meant. El Greco gave a new impact to his pictures through indigo, which separated him from the Renaissance; on his elongated noble forms, sensed out of the Spanish spirit, lay already the indigo shadows of a coming change of consciousness. In going through the indigo, one learns to overcome the ego loneliness. The ego receives stimulation and strength-ening. In this sense, one can use it with care with timid natures, together with other colours which it enhances, but also alone as a veil painting task (as shown later). The secrets of indigo, at the threshold of whose kingdom we are already now standing, are not yet to be fully apprehended but are veiled, for they reach up to the sphere of the First Heirarchy, particularly to the Thrones who, with the Spirits of Form, have created the physical earth world from the Father forces. Fear and awe can seize us, but we remember the Word. 'No man comes to the Father but by Me'; and so we will go forward through the world of indigo, through the mastery of the forces of substance, only as stronger individuals if we have taken into our hearts the forces which were brought to mankind at the Mystery of Golgotha. Fifteen hundred years after the Mystery of Golgotha, the world of indigo first emerges for mankind.

With this, the chapter on the single colours is concluded. For the therapist, the colours should be widened to World Beings, who speak their own soul language: the causes of illness lie in the soul-spiritual, and the colour world is the manifestation of this inwardness, which could otherwise remain for ever closed to outer observation.

Examples of Therapeutic Tasks

from the Course of Instruction at the School for Artistic Therapy in Boll

In this chapter, some examples will be given of how tasks can be selected for the training instruction of painting therapists in such a way, that the pupils first of all themselves experience what this kind of painting is able to bring about in the soul, if one really involves oneself in the process. Later, these experiences can be stimulations to them in their own setting of tasks. In no way, of course, does this description make any claim to completeness. The course of instruction must in addition contain very much concerning which of the different techniques—also in modelling and drawing—is suitable, considered from therapeutic points of view. Nevertheless, one is able from these examples to gain a deeper sensitivity of how to apply them, and an intuition as to which points of view are important and which are not—although today we readily overestimate some of them.

In view of the fact that many patients have never painted, it is good in the first instance to give a short introduction, in the simplest manner, to the 'wet' painting technique, and then also to Goethe's colour circle. It *Picture* is always important to go out from the whole circle, so that the colours *1* appear as a world complete in itself, yet mirroring our whole soul life again. But this introduction should not be only theoretical; one allows the pupil immediately to paint in a living way just these basic divisions, at first in the harmony of the rainbow colour sequence, but also in freer *Pictures* movement. The colour exercises should similarly be carefully painted *3-4* by the pupil, as though a patient was already looking over his shoulder. But it must be emphasised right from the beginning that nothing, absolutely nothing, which is said in this book, should be allowed to be elevated to a dogma, for occasions can always arise—and they are not even so rare—when one must do something else, because one has before one a special case, an individual human being. So there are naturally also situations where one begins with a single colour.

The pathways of colour lead the soul into the most varied moods. Each colour expresses a different soul movement, for the soul lives in the colour, she is wholly one with it, and one cannot distinguish the one from the other. The soul always voices each outer manifestation directly from the deeper level of being, and reveals outwardly her inner qualities. Through this, she creates a bridge of genuine understanding.

Picture 3 If, for example, one paints the rainbow colour sequence with veils, horizontally across the paper, with yellow in the middle, slowly passing over upwards to orange and red, and downwards through green to blue and violet, so one feels in this the tranquil image of one's own soul existence between heaven and earth, stabilised and supported by the green. One experiences at the same time one's own equilibrium in the reality of the Elements: the light-airy in the middle, beneath this, the earth-green where the light seizes the darkness and lightens it to the colour of life; below, the cooler blue which rays inwards and therefore tends to create rhythmic forms. Above, the activity is enhanced through orange into red—the picture of the spiritual impact—as far as to 'purpur' the exalted etheric red. Soul mood and the Elements blend, and I have a whole world before me. And now the journeys of discovery can begin. Here the broad field of the metamorphoses opens up, one of which was published in the article: *Painting as a Breathing Exercise* in the *Städtlerbriefen*. A separate leaflet with these explanations and with pictures is obtainable from the School.

It is important that right from the beginning, the pupil is induced to experience the colours as a World-element around him, to place himself wholly within them, and through this to feel how in Nature, the pictures of the times of day and the yearly seasons are moods of the World-earth-soul, in which the Sun, as the World Ego, stimulates breathing *Pictures 22-25* life. The last chapter of the first volume of *Zur Künstlerische Therapie* deals with the healing forces which a living with the times of the year can bestow. To what is said there, it should be further mentioned that the seasons of the year represent a kind of incarnation of the light. The spring experience begins with the experience of the change 'in the air', the light returns, it ensouls the air, the plants so to speak drink it in and create the green which is wholly filled with light, they elaborate it to the living carbohydrate—light which has become substance. The light lives on in the plants, the green becomes darker and heavier, until in the autumn the light releases in the fire its flaming colours. Then autumn leaves us behind in the darkness of winter, and the trees stand there with their skeleton-like, bare trunks and branches. Again it is a picture of how our imperishable immortal being plunges into the material world, and ever and again returns to the world of reality, 'eternally changing', as in Goethe's poem about the water: 'From heaven it comes, to heaven it ascends, and to earth it must again descend, eternally changing'. We should learn to read much more in Mother Nature, for she makes us healthy. If one has first painted all the Elements, then one can practise each Element singly, and in elaborating, can lay the emphasis on the most varied matters, either on the colour movement—calm or dramatic—or on the transitions—slow or quick—or on the strength of the colour. These are all elements which in therapy one must later observe and aim to employ, in order to stimulate the corresponding process in the soul.

These exercises, carefully carried out, always satisfy, because they correspond to an inner reality. So one now allows the Elements to produce with one another the most varied Nature phenomena or Nature moods. Fire, water, air and earth appear, and one conjures them all from out of the rainbow. Through this, the sketches lose the arbitrary, intellectual, thought-out quality, the abstract fixedness. The brush stroke will follow imitatively the movement of the Elements. The magic word is 'to identify oneself'. One must become water right into the fingertips when one paints water, breathing with it as waves of the sea or as a rushing waterfall, dashing against the rocks as breakers, and at last solidifying to ice.

Pictures 5-12

Then follows the coming-into-being of the plants. In the darkness of the earth in-streaming light brings out the green (Goethe: Blue and yellow unite themselves downwards to green), and this grows upwards as plant beings until the light-cosmos sets the blossoms on fire with all colours. These tasks with the plants will at first be carried out as a simple enhancement of yellow to a red blossom, which nightly passes over into sleep in blueness, and then also with their metamorphoses between the seed in darkness, the roots and leaves, blossoms and fruit. All this awakens the inclination for perception and observation above all in the plant world, which shows the etheric life-processes in purity. The whole plant kingdom is a precipitate of the world of life; the plant kingdom shapes itself from the laws and possibilities of the etheric formative forces. Dr Hilmar Walter gives a specially graphic description in her valuable book: *Die Pflanzenwelt, ihre Verwandtschaft zur Erden- und Menschheitsentwicklung.* The plant kingdom corresponds in the macrocosm to the etheric nature of the human body, which mediates between the inwardness of the soul, and the environment. As we enclose ourselves with our skin, so the Earth-organism envelops itself with the living plant covering, which is its sense-organ for the Sun forces of the cosmos. In the physical world, the plant has only one physical and one etheric body; but observed spiritually, it is beamed upon from all sides by cosmic-astral Star forces, which bring it about that the whole rainbow appears in the colours of the blossoms; also that the plants grow spirally from stipule to stipule, that the trees form leaf crowns, and still much more. I would like to quote Dr Walter with regard to this. The therapist should deepen his connection with Nature through spiritual science, and through a higher knowledge, enliven in himself the significance of the simple. In this sense, the following explanations may be quoted:

Pictures 13-17

Corresponding to the seven main planets, seven Group-souls can also be fundamentally distinguished in the plant world, and these forces work together with the Group Egos of the plants. These are descendants of the Spirits of Wisdom, of the leaders of the Old Sun development, who also gave to the human being, from their own substance, the foundation of his etheric body. They work from the sun towards us. We have the direction of their forces if we unite the sun with the middle point of the earth. They give to the plant stem the direction which acts towards the middle point of the earth. There in the middle point of the earth, they have the centre-point of their being, and in their totality, form the Ego of the Earth-organism. To this also comes the activity of the Spirits of the rotation periods, as descendants of the beings of the First Hierarchy. They regulate the time changes—the succession of the seasons, the alternation of day and night. They are also those who bring about through fertilisation, the connection between the activity of the Spirits of Movement and the Spirits of Wisdom, in that they regulate those organs which follow the spiral movements of the planets, or are arranged circularly, as the stamens; but the stem growth reaches its conclusion in the ovary.

We have almost completely lost the living relationship to Nature which still existed in the Middle Ages, when she was revered as the goddess Natura. We receive her phenomena as if the World-All were really only a calculating machine directed by physical forces. But if spiritual thoughts about the plants live in the mind of the therapist, these act in a healing manner without their being expressed. The therapist will also be better able to find, for each kind of thinking or soul mood of the patients, the adequate artistic expression of the task, in order to bring something from the heavenly world which surrounds us as plant pictures, to the soul of the sick person. The taking of such pains always works so as to cause the depressed forces of the etheric body to blossom. One therefore paints the plants, and in particular the flowers, in the way that Rudolf Steiner recommended for the Waldorf school-children of approximately nine and ten years old, that is: 'so that they appear animated'. The teaching about the plants should, in addition, always be dealt with in connection with the life of the earth as a unified organism. Often the expression of a single sentence in this direction during the painting is sufficient to open a door.

Pictures 18-19

The trees are the lungs of the earth. They enliven the whole fluid-organism through the enormous stream of evaporation, which again leads the water upwards, in order that it may fall again, in its circular course, as fertilising rain. The woods are a climatic factor of the first importance. The single tree in its uprightness, its closed form-character being always a picture of the human individuality, stands in a similar way between heaven and earth, spreads its arms lovingly over a space, and is able to grant shelter, as though the tree would invite friends here. Poetry knows how to sing of this:

59

At the well before the gate, there stands a linden tree,
I dreamt in its shadow so many sweet dreams.
Am Brunnen vor dem Tore, da steht ein Lindenbaum,
Ich träumt in seinem Schatten so manchen süssen Traum...

In this song, both the whole soul-wealth of the true Romantic Movement, as well as the real being of the tree in relation to the human ego, are grasped simultaneously in an ingenuous way. It is the destiny-carrying quality of the ego which sees itself reflected. The tree stands in wind and weather, in snow and in the glow of the sun, as a lovely birch in the valley, or as a weather-beaten mountain pine at a great height, meeting the lightning without total destruction and still blooming again with new life from out of the ruins.

It is interesting that in our time of misunderstanding of the ego, hardly anyone who lives in a big city, patient or pupil, really understands the tree. He paints a 'paint brush' or a 'big head', and only after some time do rhythm and breathing come into it—light and shadow, the striving heavenwards and the being rooted in the earth—through which the tree becomes a creation of the middle region, and acquires a *Picture* form which is full of character and which has a genuine skeleton, whose *25* gesture becomes visible in winter.

There is still, in painting, a special means by which to express the turning of the soul outwards in the deed through the will, in contrast to the self-communion and the turning inwards. This happens through consideration of both the new ideas: 'lustre' and 'image' in Rudolf Steiner's colour teaching. The colours blue, red, and yellow are 'lustre' colours, because they have an outward-streaming will character; the colours black, white, peach-blossom, and green have an 'image' character, which means that they are shaded down to 'image'. The more exact spiritual-scientific foundation can be gleaned from the book: *Das Wesen der Farbe* by Rudolf Steiner. Instead of theorising about this, one may look at the two small portraits which depict in an artistic way a fiery, outwards-turning character, and a person with quiet inwardness. These two sketches speak for themselves.

Pictures Then there follows for the prospective therapist a study of the animal *20-21* forms. These are not ego forms as in the case of the human being, but each is a soul quality which has become form—that is, an astral form. *Pictures* One sees best in contour, in profile, what is characteristic in an animal. *26-29* With the human being also, the silhouette exhibits more of his quality of soul, while the ego reveals itself when one looks at the human form face to face, and is able to meet the glance.

The animals are in a certain dependence upon their geographical habitat, and will therefore be painted in their landscape, and sensed out of the mood of the landscape, not abstractly drawn in and then coloured. Experience shows that this period gives much opportunity, in a group, for a liberating cheerfulness. The animals so quickly acquire human traits, and the effort to represent them calls forces of sympathy to the fore. The Group Egos of the animals are cosmic beings, and throughout the olden cultures were still looked upon as portraits of the deities. The human being has the totality of the plant forces in his etheric body, as well as the whole animal kingdom in his astral body, but comprehended as a unity and humanised through the ego. But in many a corner of his worldwide soul, he still has a kinship to an animal. Expressed pictorially: the process of humanising is not yet completed. St Francis, it is true, preached to all animals that in the World Ego of the Representative of Mankind, they should find their Lord and Master, who understands how to soften their wild nature; but nevertheless sometimes a cock crows or a gull laughs, a wolf howls or a bull bellows. If the ego stands above that, then here humour can begin which, as is well known, includes an 'even though'.

When the kingdoms of Nature have been passed through, the human being in his free activity must also be formed out of movement, preferably in one of his basic professions as a hunter, a breeder of animals, a farmer or a fisherman—there are of course also other examples. Again it will be a question of the movement being sensed from within, so that in this way the pupil first brings out the gesture and forms it from this sensing, and not from outside. A colour movement first appears, out of which the figure is condensed. Here, it is over and over again made evident whether, through divining of his own form, a person can discover the human proportions. The guidance towards the human form through these exercises is usually preceded at an earlier time by a reflection upon oneself through the task of forming a blue space, and placing oneself within it. This exercise has something very calming in it and leads to a quiet composure through the blue. As a veiling task, this

Pictures 30-31

exercise acquires in addition the overtone of a gentle freeing from the unrest of daily life in a dignified world of blue, as lustre of the soul. But so that one does not remain fixed in the blue space, the task will be continued to a meeting with red within the blue space. Blue—so it is said in Rudlof Steiner's colour teaching—draws lilac, reddish-blue, after it; red, on the other hand, drives orange, yellow and green before it. Thus through the meeting, the whole colour circle appears as an artistic sketch. If one follows such laws, even if it is only in artistic, free treatment, then one experiences a considerable quickening of expression. The meeting, the turning of the red towards the blue, becomes real, and does not remain a cool confrontation. It is the soul-warmth which creates such transitions, and which also then comes to expression in the picture. The 'artistic' consists in this, that such hints, indicated in a free manner, are not painted in an abstract intellectual way because one knows of this relationship. On a higher plane, colours are real beings. Because the human spirit forms them on the earthly plane, it does not need to allow them their own wills. Rudolf Steiner calls one's attention

61

to this in commenting upon the image and lustre colours. One is able as a painter, for instance, to transform an image colour into lustre, or a lustre colour into image. With blue, for example, whose lustre nature would like to become lighter towards the centre—if one spreads it out evenly, as does Fra Angelico, then one has transformed the lustre nature into the quiet image nature; and this blue is then the picture of the depths of the soul, in which the religious contents live—which Fra Angelico represents. In the blue space, one can in addition verify that the soul-mood immediately loses the elevated romantic overtone, if the base is transformed with yellow veils to green; then one is immediately in well-established earthly consciousness. Or, if blue is enhanced to violet, one observes how the dreamy mood deepens to lonely seclusion, and yet is also a turning towards the Divine. The free manifestation of the whole rainbow in the meeting with red is, on the other hand, a healthy phenomenon of the middle region. These exercises are preliminary studies for the illustraion of fairy tales, fables and legends, which play a special role in the training, beginning with the simplest childlike form right up to the conscious, carefully formed veil picture.

A few general examples will now be described, and indications given in pictures, of how one expresses artistically, special therapeutically applied processes, or how one can 'clothe' them; because it is in the first place a question of the contrast between a predominance of the forces of the upper astral body in the direction of sclerosis and as far as a swelling, or of the lower astral body in the direction of inflammation and loosening—in both cases, after the failure of the ego-organisation. For this, there are the tasks of contour-loosening for the first case, and of the creation of structure, and forming in the second case. The loosening can begin, for example, with a sharply contoured reproduction, for which purpose any suitable copy will serve (we generally choose Macke *Pictures* or Marc). This will then be 'dissolved' in two or three stages. Many *32-34* people find this task astonishingly difficult; it is as though only the contour could give them a standpoint or firm basis. The loosening then leads quickly to a colour-chaos instead of to the consistent tracing back to the colour-harmony. If this happens, it is instructive and interesting to consider the process backwards, in order to discover how a picture really forms itself slowly from out of the colour, until the colours mutually limit each other and through this, the contour arises, which did not previously of itself exist. With this, one is within the painting method for the future which Rudolf Steiner characterised with the words: 'Paint from out of the colour'. First one paints only the colour mood, and then out of this, a picture is condensed.

On the other hand, faulty shaping forces can be improved through the following structural tasks. One again takes a reproduction, preferably from the pre-Renaissance or Renaissance periods, because in that time, composition was especially developed. The picture of one's choice will then be covered with transparent paper and on this, the most important points of the picture are connected, producing a structure-drawing. One can take as motif, gestures, the direction of the glance, architecture, or still other elements, so that the most varied constructions can arise. These tasks were already carried out earlier in the Arlesheim Clinic, and originated with Anni Ruthenberg who in the 1930s worked artistically with patients in the Clinic, mainly with modelling; but above all, she cared for them spiritually through the communal study of spiritual-scientific lectures. Through tasks which came near to geometrical construction, she drew attention to the fact that in most cases, the basic forms of the four kinds of etheric forces are as follows: the circle for the warmth-ether, the triangle for the light-ether, the half-moon for the sound or chemical-ether, and the square for the life-ether. The picure is then generally a woven unity of such basic forms. Of course, other curves and forms can also appear, because it should be a free search for the structural element. This task is interesting by reason of the fact that the patient gets to know, and gets to know well, many a picture; and that in spite of the structural element, one feels oneself still to be within the domain of artistic freedom. Nevertheless, the soul-spiritual will already be called upon from out of the colour-sphere of feeling by the formative conceptual region of the head. One finds oneself at the transition to pure geometrical drawing.

Geometry was recommended by Rudolf Steiner for purely inflammatory, 'liquefying' illness-situations, such as we perhaps find with tuberculosis or osteomyelitis. Here generally the inclination of the patient comes to meet—from a healthy instinct—the therapeutic-artistic process. But it can also be that just such sick people like to repeat their illness-process on the painting paper. Then no form is forthcoming. That does no harm, if it is recognised and its transformation is immediately worked upon. It depends on the therapist as to whether he can make the desired task palatable and pleasing or not.

Pictures 35-40
Now come further special exercises to serve as examples for soul-movements which one wishes to stimulate: Again in the first instance, such contrasts as narrowness and breadth, or a thunderstorm and the subsequent clearing up, or waking and sleeping. Such exercises naturally bring about a deepened soul-breathing. The expansion of the self, and its drawing together, is the purpose of these exercises. In the accompanying examples, the interior of the woods as 'narrowness', and the peace of the evening as 'breadth', speak for themselves, and likewise the darkness of the storm, and the sunny stillness afterwards. For waking and sleeping, the warm earth-brown is chosen for waking, with two people wandering over the Good Earth. When sleep comes, one draws over the brown picture a 'purpur' veil from above downwards, and then that dreamy imaginative mood is obtained which gives quality and depth even to the simplest production. Here, 'purpur' is able to enter

into its special rights, for it stands at the border of the invisible, of the spiritual, into which we plunge in sleep. The sun, which we follow with the spirit-soul in the day and night rhythm, comes and goes with 'purpur'.

One is reminded by painting with 'purpur' of a task which Rudolf Steiner suggested for the upper classes of the Waldof School, namely, to copy Rembrandt in the same kind of way. Burnt sienna rises from below upwards, to serve for the form of the picture; then from above downwards, 'purpur' is laid on to deepen the artistic mood and finally, a quite delicate yellow is applied to the lightest places. It is astonishing how nearly, in this way, one approaches to the spiritual quality of Rembrandt's work, even if in the original, still other colours appear. This triad represents a cosmic-earthly balance, within which the ego, along with the delicate yellow, places itself.

Pictures 41-42

A further task for the uplifting and encouragement of the ego of a dejected personality is the 'upward glance to the heights'. Again and again a sick person is met with, who rarely lifts his gaze from the ground. They lose through this the freedom of the surroundings, which one experiences with such deep delight on a mountain summit. Therefore this summit region must first appear in consciousness as a goal, not to be physically climbed, but as a stage which the earth builds for the feet of the Gods.

An older humanity which was connected with Nature knew that there above in the inaccessible, Hierarchical beings weave around the peaks, and that these are really Castles of the Gods; they therefore always enjoyed veneration and created pious feelings. This is not at all so long ago, so that we possess some evidence about it. Certainly in later times, the human being has conquered these peaks also. He should take possession of the earth, but not as an arrogant opponent of the Gods, not in that mood which Rudolf Steiner—looking forwards to the end of the century—expressed with the words: 'impudent cocksureness'. Rather, the countenance of the earth should become a sublime parable to him, one of the noblest works of art of Divine Nature. It can only promote health—when for brief moments we glance up from our daily work or from our worries—if we lift up our feeling to the fair heights of these virgin peaks. Here art verges on religion, and both act in a stimulating way on the human etheric body.

Pictures 42-45

The true soul nourishment in a narrower sense for people who have become dried-up, quite prosaic and lacking in fantasy, is to be found in the fairy tales. That which milk signifies for the small child, fairy tales represent for the soul of the human being, who should retain forces of childhood during his whole life. The world of technology, which yokes us and encloses us in a web, makes the world empty and barren, hard and unfeeling. The tendencies to such illness-causing soul-situations are alarmingly evident to our perception, and both therapy and prophylaxis can be created out of art.

The genuine fairy tales lead us back into the past before our birth. Many speak in pictures about life before birth, and of the path of the soul to the earth in incarnation (Little Brother and Little Sister, Snow White, Hansel and Gretel, and so on). This path is full of dangers, there are always tasks to be fulfilled, and the higher being belonging to each one to be attained—prince and princess are our own higher soul-spiritual being. Fairy tales satisfy the depths of the soul through their true content, even when the understanding is only artistic, and sometimes not even that. But in the depths, the upbuilding forces of childhood are active, and the consciousness of our own situation on the earth dawns upon us. The method of the fairy tale theme lies so rightly in the domain of the play impulse, in the sense in which Schiller described it, as that sphere where we are fully human—neither restricted by laws nor driven by egoistic passions or desires. In so far as we move freely through all transformations, we equip ourselves to overcome, by means of our ego, all dangers on the path as does the prince, who is helped by the animals and the Elemental beings, if his heart is pure. Genuine fairy tales cannot be invented intellectually; in bygone days they have been intuitively perceived and derive from the Sages. Artistically, they should be executed wholly in the 'wet' painting technique of the Waldorf School. With this, there is first a colour mood, out of which the appropriate figures condense, if possible in rich colours. Each patient may paint quite naively, as though he is still a child. In therapy, it is never a question of perfectionism, but of the activity as such, of the accompanying soul-movement and of the resultant satisfaction and joy, for these are the most health-giving forces of the soul. That does not mean that this sentence is to be taken superficially and trivially. Also, healing often proceeds through crises, but the patient must sense that he follows a meaningful path which has a worthwhile goal.

The process of painting itself works in the soul, in that the two basic forces, sympathy and antipathy, are brought into a lively interplay. Each new feeling is like a source of strength, it emerges in the soul as an impulse, which pulsates and continues to vibrate in the soul for a longer or shorter period. In the direction of sympathy lies the turning towards the will, which ascends right into the senses and would like to grasp the world. In the direction of antipathy lies the keeping of one's distance, the 'onlooker' awareness and artistic judgement. This colourful swinging to and fro 'moistens' the soul which has become dry and barren, and new, healthier soul-movement can flourish. The damage—still not at all foreseen and widely underestimated—which is caused by the radio and television is not only soul-spiritual in the generalisation of judgements and de-personalisation, but also physical in that eye and ear become ever more insensitive. Through this is also prepared an ever stronger isolation of the individual within his own concerns, in that he becomes more difficult to approach, and mass-opinion cheerfully 'steam-rollers' everyone who thinks differently and spreads an unsocial atmosphere. Here also it is necessary to find the Measure, and to recognise the nature of the modern culture-media. Fanaticism, even in the rejection of these media, is not in place, but a conscious handling and above all, a 'seeing through' them.

In order to strengthen the ego in the present-day technological world, where awakeness in the senses is a demand of the times, one can, in the artistic field, use indigo. Its nature is fully described in the chapter on the single colours. The task—in order to draw the ego right into the senses—is a representation of a city picture, or of a factory or a techno-*Picture* logical milieu, as a veil painting picture purely in indigo. The vertically
47 placed picture will be created in such a way that one begins with large veils; and through slow graduation into smaller veils, a composition is produced which arises through an intrinsic continuous process of division. It is known in pedagogy that in calculation, Rudolf Steiner has assigned division to the ego. Other aspects of calculation belong to different members of the human being. The example shows that this task can of course be freely handled, and it immensely stimulates the fantasy to add still more small details. Thereby the whole picture remains in a transparent, artistic, elevated style of painting, showing this dead world in a kind of transfigured lightness. Again the ego stands at the boundary of the colour world, without however forsaking it, so that one can at any time add quite fine shades of other colours. This one cannot do with black/white drawing.

If one now wants to lead over into colour from black/white, there are various transcriptions of a black/white picture into a self-chosen colour mood. The burden of the composition is taken away, and the patient is able to devote himself to the mood and ensoul the picture with colour in the most varied ways. This can of course also be done with a colour-ed reproduction. Then it becomes a transcription with a greater copying *Picture* aspect. To this it may be added, that a small reproduction can be con-
46 siderably enlarged, without measuring but purely by the judgement of the eye. Judgement by the eye gives evidence of the presence of the ego in the seeing-process. The enlarging means that the etheric body must itself expand. These exercises are also carried out by pupils with special appreciation. With patients, one allows some simplification—in fact, one frankly asks for it. The perpetual association with our technological surroundings presses the etheric body strongly into the physical, so that free movement in forming becomes difficult; and in painting, a repetition of the same thing in stiff form sets in. Through copying, the pupil learns to know all the possibilities of form which a Master, and not he himself, has created. Side by side with the enlargements and transcriptions, copying therefore also plays an important role in the training. In an earlier time, painting was first learnt chiefly through imitation; that

was the case for all the arts. Already very early, one went to a Master in order to watch or to listen, or to imitate his movements, before producing work of one's own. But also, a fair copy lovingly executed arouses slumbering capacities, it creates appetite, encourages, and in addition gives a surer foundation to the timid.

Pictures 48-50

Later, there are again other tasks to awaken the capacity for the composition or harmonising and forming of small coloured areas, which are first put spontaneously on the paper. It is certainy acknowledged, for example, that with a ruined wall, Leonardo da Vinci practised imagining a whole battle from its shadow-patches, that is, he created a composition. We also practise something similar in miniature with sick people. One cannot be sufficiently inventive in order to maintain a lively interest in the artistic possibilities. A bouquet of flowers can be created from the small coloured patches, or a circus, or yet many other motifs, from soft gradations to dramatic contrasts of colour; but at the end, everything should appear gathered up into a uniform mood, preferably a cheerful one.

This is of course only a small section of the work which will be practised throughout the year and for still longer. But it can be inferred from this that the practising of artistic therapy is a profession which claims the whole of a person's strength, if it is grasped in its breadth and depth, and that it can only be developed on a spiritual-scientific foundation. It is obvious that many questions still remain open, and many hints by Rudolf Steiner have not yet been considered. It is most important that each prospective therapist should study the Waldorf School artistic programme, and should himself work through in painting what corresponds in technique and content to the different age stages. Likewise, the history of art is important in connection with the development of the different members of the human being and of the soul. This is also the content of special periods at the School. Modelling, and the graphic possibilities for therapy, still remain completely untouched. An intensive study of the paintings from the first Goetheanum constitutes the crowning point of the training. The foundation-stone of this building was laid while Mercury stood as evening star in the Scales. The task of this buiding for mankind really could not be more clearly expressed in the language of the stars. Mercury as evening star is the leader of the souls on the path to a new cosmic connection, to contact with the World Soul, and to an understanding of the spiritual background of the world. From this direction, the impulses must come in the future which are able to contribute to the healing of mankind.

Raphael-Mercury

Since olden times, medical science has stood under the Sign of Mercury. Already in Egyptian times he was known as Hermes-Thoth, the three-times wise inaugurator of Egyptian culture. The Egyptians had the task of bringing down the heavenly dimensions and of transforming them into earthly measure. Mercury, who later in Greek times was the messenger of the gods, mediated this. He was therefore also the teacher in the Egyptian Mysteries. In Thoth, Mercury was venerated as the morning star, which went in advance of the sun, and thus—even if under another name—of the Christ Sun, which had so to speak sent him in advance, before his Guiding Spirit descended to the earth at the Turning Point of Time. Mercury as evening star was Anubis, who conducted and weighed the Dead, and who followed the sun in the evening into the spiritual, invisible world—in the language of the Egyptians: when the Barque of the Sun travels back at night under the earth towards the dawn. The Greeks also knew both phases of Mercury in Hermes, the winged messenger of the gods, and Hermes Psychopompos, who likewise conducted the Dead. With his Snake-staff, which Zeus once bestowed on him, he could lull to sleep and awaken, that is to say, he could loosen the soul from the body and again reunite it. This is the function that makes him into the administrator of health, this being the right measure of incarnation of the soul in the physical-etheric body. The rhythmical function of the breathing, regulated by a sun rhythm, carries into us the health-giving forces, the healing forces. Every illness is a displacement of the balance of forces in the sense either of a predominance of the in-breathing (the astral body plunges in too deeply, binding and hardening), or of the out-breathing (this impulse of the astral body, which stimulates the etheric body from within, loosens too strongly and causes inflammation). A symbol such as the Staff of Mercury naturally has many meanings: but always the two snakes are pictures of the astral body climbing around the Ego-staff, by which the astral forces are kept in balance—that is the forces of predilection and sympathy, or of alienation antipathy. We need both forces, the first at the pole of the will, and the second in the sense-nerve system, where it frees itself.

At the time of the Egyptian Mysteries, there was a deeper knowledge of the cosmic forces forming the human being. Hermes was known as 'three-times wise' because he possessed the wisdom of the Zodiac, the Planets, and the Elements. In

Greece, only the wisdom of the Elements existed, and then that also slowly disappeared when Hippocrates closed the Temple, and thereafter earthly substances were more and more utilised as remedies.

The metal mercury is the only one which is fluid, remaining mobile also in its physical manifestation; it has a deep connection to warmth and to fire, as no transformation is possible entirely without warmth. The noblest representation of the Resurrection out of the Fire was in the Phoenix Mysteries in Asia Minor, in Arabia, the land of the Queen of Sheba, and in Phoenicia—these were also Mercury Mysteries. Mercury, on its path through the heavens—continually plunging into the sun's fire in its conjunctions with the sun, and its unceasing brilliant emergence—is really the archetype of this myth. One knows today that Phoenix coins were minted, when Mercury stood in front of the Sun, in those countries where these Phoenix Mysteries prevailed.

But if we now turn to Central Europe, then one must say that the German folk were already in early times brought up with a Mercury spirit. It was Wotan, the Wanderer, roaring in the storm, accompanied by his Spirits of the Fallen—the warriors who had fallen on the battlefield, the most courageous, who lived with him in Valhalla. He who brings the trees—the lungs of the earth—to rustle in the wind, also moves our lungs in the breath-stream, and thus carries the spirit downwards into the blood; Thor with his hammer is the picture of the pulse, who accompanies Wotan. Thor, as Rudolf Steiner recounted, was the most powerful Angel to be at any time venerated; he carries the sun-rhythm into the blood. He has the iron-Mars character, and is through this related to Michael, who with his sword of cosmic iron restrains the sulphur nature of the dragon in the blood. With this, the ego-man is born, the individuality draws into the physical body. The Creation of the Gods is completed; and in the tragic art of the Twilight of the Gods is revealed the world-historic fact, that from now onwards man becomes responsible for his own future destiny and for that of the earth.

In olden times, Mercury was considered to be also the Revealer of Destiny. We experience destiny in the feeling human being of the middle region, where the transformations take place, the essential development-decisions. Speech detaches itself from the inner soul; to the speech organism belongs everything which the breath stream forms in the out-breathing, from the diaphragm as the basis of resonance right up to the tip of the tongue. The god Wotan is deeply involved with the development of speech and of intelligence. He brings the wisdom of the Runes, and 'advising' is succeeded by 'thinking'.

The Mercury force must keep the life of processes in us fluid; the breathing must penetrate the whole organism right into the smallest cell, for should it suffocate, or suffer the contrary—that the breathing destroys the cell—then we are in one way or another ill. Mercury-Raphael secretes the health-giving forces within our breathing system. Rudolf Steiner has revealed to us that the same hierarchical being whom people of old revered under the name of Mercury, is called in the Christian wisdom of Dionysius Areopagita, Raphael. Since the Mystery of Golgotha, the Archangel Raphael administers the cosmic healing forces, and leads them through the breathing function into the rhythmical human being.

The human soul-spirit, which from time to time comes into incarnation, is today entirely individual. Through earth experience and destiny, it has much connected with it which will not be of value for eternity, but is the result of the so-called Fall of Man, and originates from egoistic desires. All this is the source of our illnesses and of death, and prevents us from building up a healthy body. The human being will at some future time develop higher to Freedom and Love, and will find his way back to his Divine origin and archetype, but today we are not yet so mature. Every misused freedom, every unkindness, will create a new, sorrowful trial of destiny. But since the Mystery of Golgotha, Raphael-Mercury is our quiet companion, in the same way that he once accompanied Tobias, and at each stage of our long path he brings us the healing forces which we need. While we are in the earthly body, he unites us again with the cosmic Sun forces. The human ego must seize these forces and give to each deed a Mercurial—that is, a therapeutic—character; this must happen actively in the future. Everything that Rudolf Steiner, together with Ita Wegman, inaugurated on the basis of an extended Art of Healing through Spiritual Science, is likewise pertinent to the strengthening of these Mercury forces in the human being, activating spiritual-creativity and leading the soul back to the source of her cosmic union with Nature. This happens in the medical field both through the new way of preparing the medicines, and especially also through artistic therapy, which calls the ego, the spirit, on to the earthly plane. If one describes the Archangel Michael as the 'Countenance of Christ', because through him the Sun-strength speaks, and he administers the Cosmic Intelligence, so one could say of Raphael that he works in the Sun-breathing of the Christ, and through him, the Christ's healing breath blows about us.

Bibliography

Rudolf Steiner   *Occult Science - an Outline.* Rudolf Steiner Press, London, 1984.

Speech and Drama. Rudolf Steiner Press, London, 1959.

Art as Seen in the Light of Mystery Wisdom. Rudolf Steiner Press, London, 1984.

The Arts and their Mission. Anthroposophic Press, New York, 1964.

The Four Seasons and the Archangels. Rudolf Steiner Press, London, 1984

The Wisdom of Man, of the Soul, and of the Spirit. Anthroposophy, Psychosophy, Pneumatosophy. Anthroposophic Press, New York, 1971.

Colour. Rudolf Steiner Press, London, 1982.

Rudolf Steiner and Ita Wegman   *Fundamentals of Therapy. An Extension of the Art of Healing through Spiritual Science.* Rudolf Steiner Press, London, 1983.

M. Hauschka   *Rhythmical Massage as indicated by Ita Wegman.* Rudolf Steiner Press, London, 1979.

Not translated into English:

Rudolf Steiner   *Das Wesen der Künste.*
Kunst und Kunsterkenntnis.
Das Wesen der Farben.
Wessen bedarf die Menschheit zur Neugestaltung der Menschheit.

Ita Wegman   *Im Anbruch des Wirkens für eine Erweiterung der Heilkunst.* Natura Verlag.

W. Bühler   *Nordlicht, Blitz und Regenbogen.* Philosophisch-Anthroposophischer Verlag.

L. Eberhard   *Heilkräfte der Farben.* Drei Eichen Verlag.

H. Frieling   *Mensch und Farbe.* Heyne Verlag.

M. Hauschka   *Zur Künstlerischen Therapie, Band I.* Verlag Schule für Künstlerische Therapie und Massage.

W. Kaelin   *Krebsfrühdiagnose - Krebsvorbeugung.* Vittorio Klostermann Verlag.

H. Walter   *Die Pflanzenwelt, ihre Verwandtschaft zur Erden- und Menschheitsentwicklung.* Natura Verlag.

Examples from the
Course of Instruction
at the
School for Artistic Therapie
at Boll

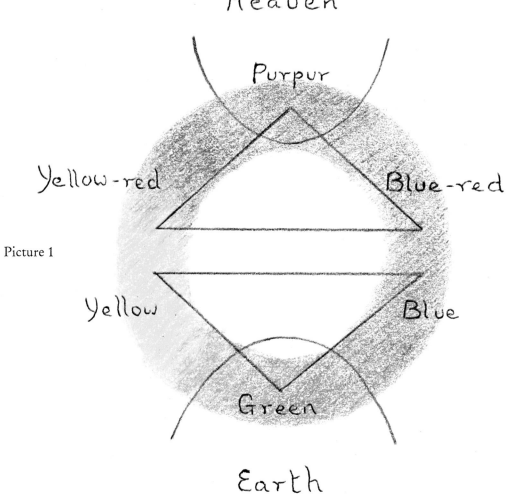

Heaven

Purpur

Yellow-red

Blue-red

Picture 1

Yellow

Blue

Green

Earth

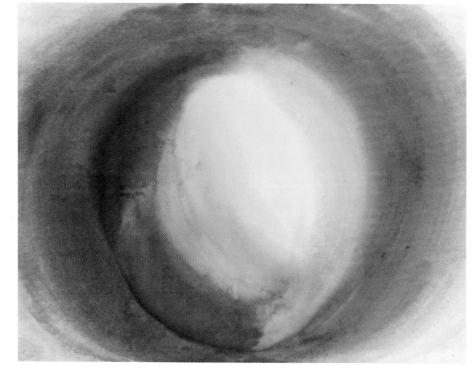

Picture 2

Picture 3

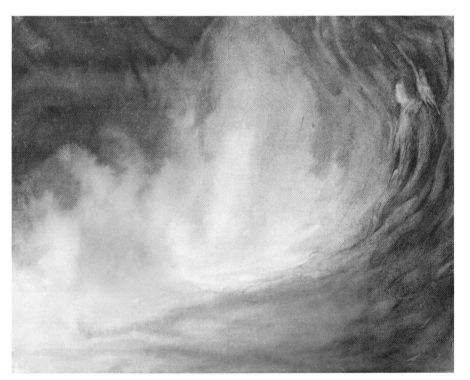

Picture 4

Picture 5

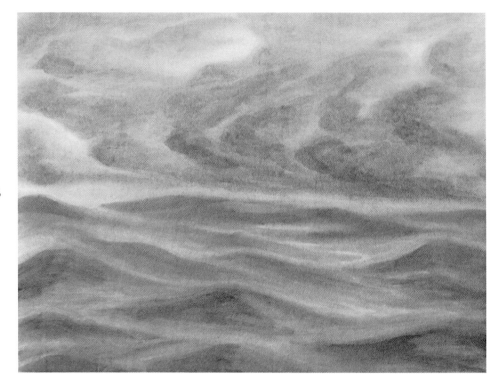

Picture 6

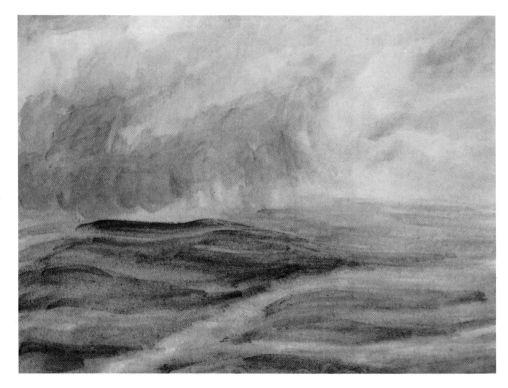

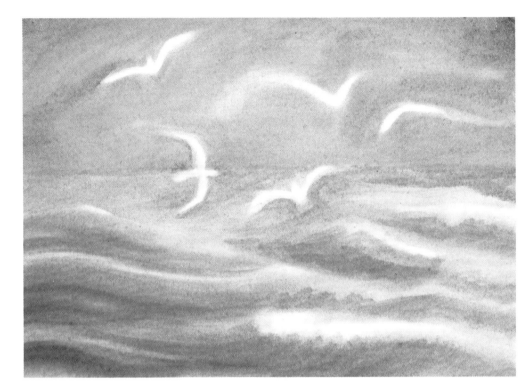

Picture 7

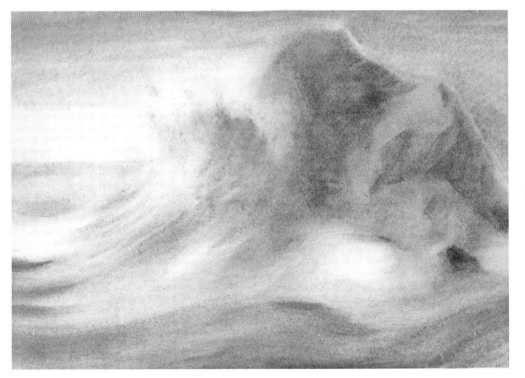

Picture 8

Picture 9

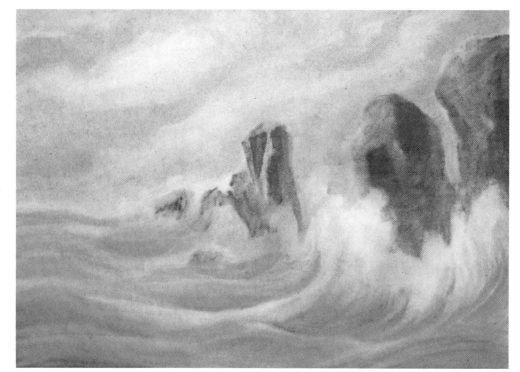

Picture 10

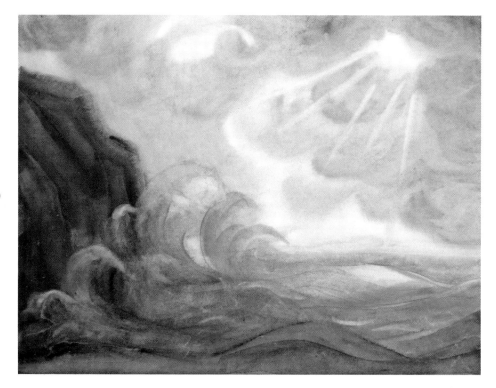

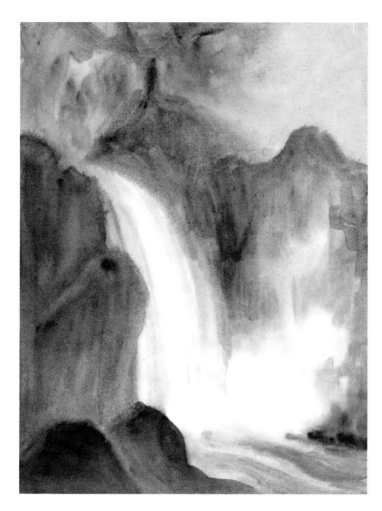

Picture 11

Picture 12

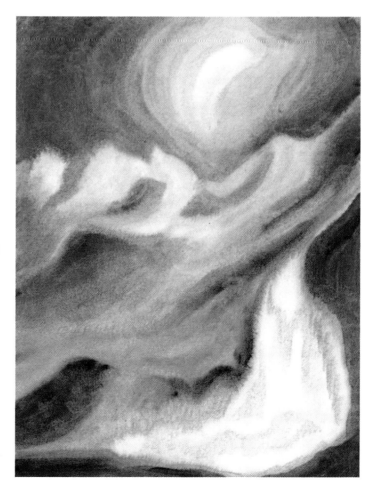

Picture 13

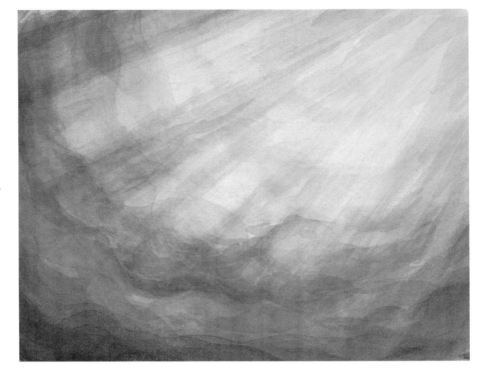

Picture 14

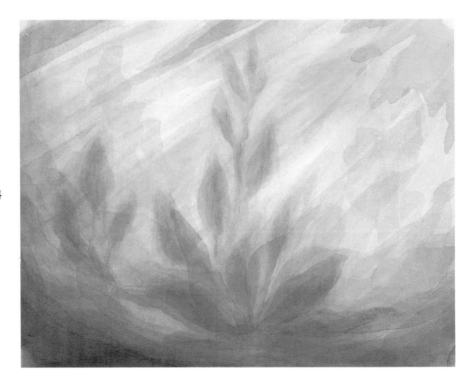

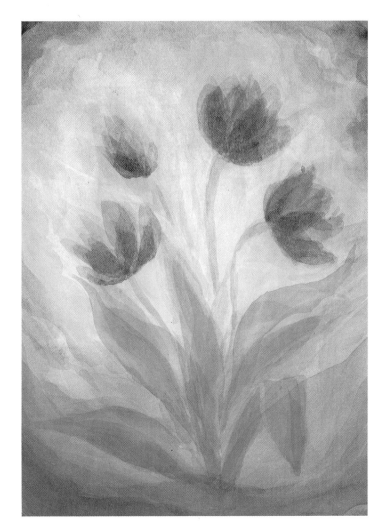

Picture 15

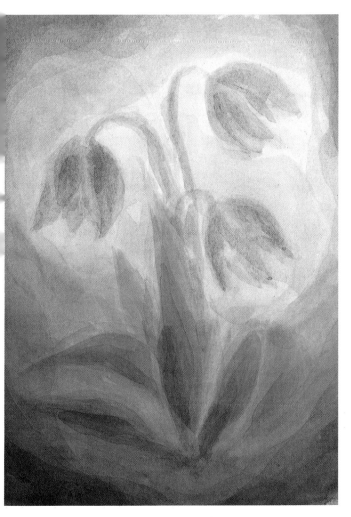

Picture 16

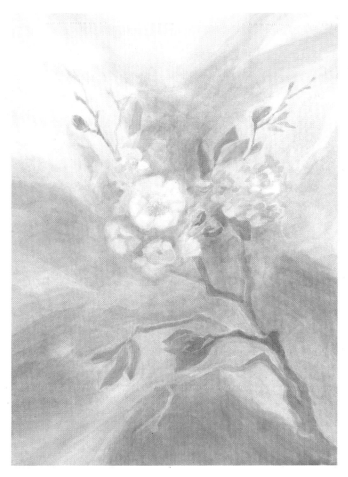

Picture 17

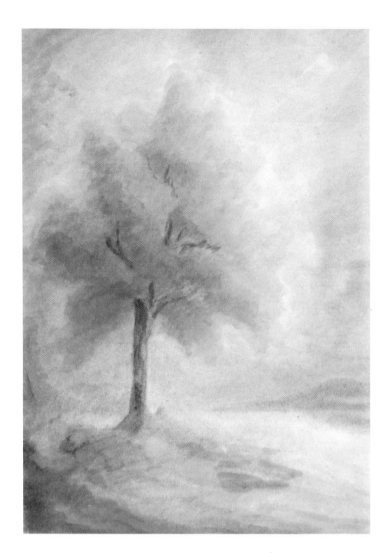

Picture 18

Picture 19

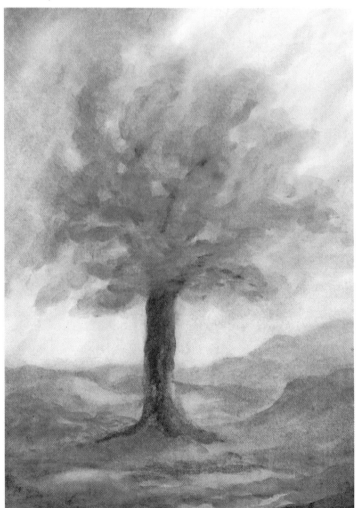

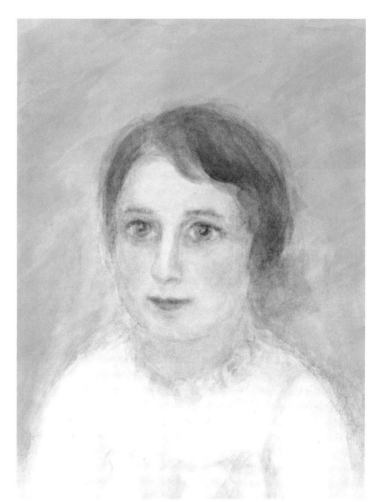

Picture 20

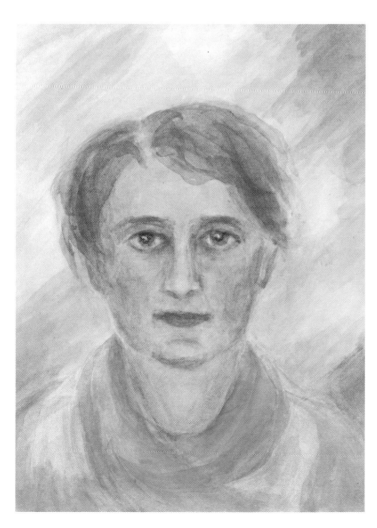

Picture 21

Picture 22

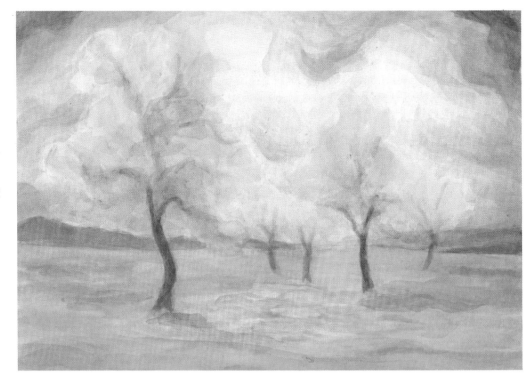

Picture 23

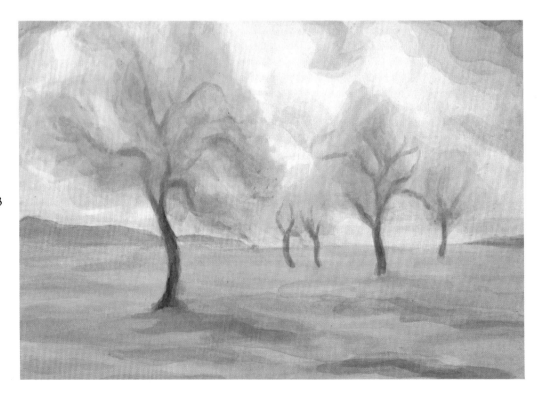

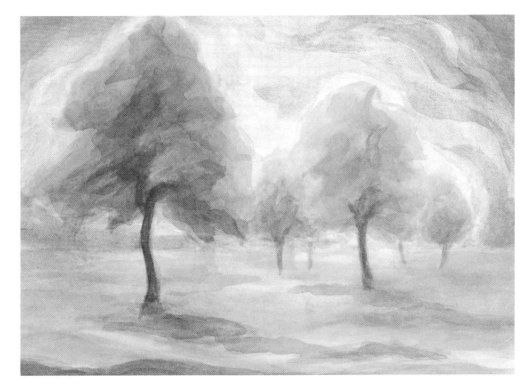

Picture 24

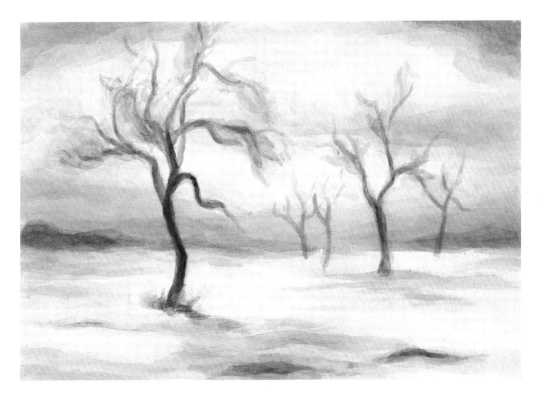

Picture 25

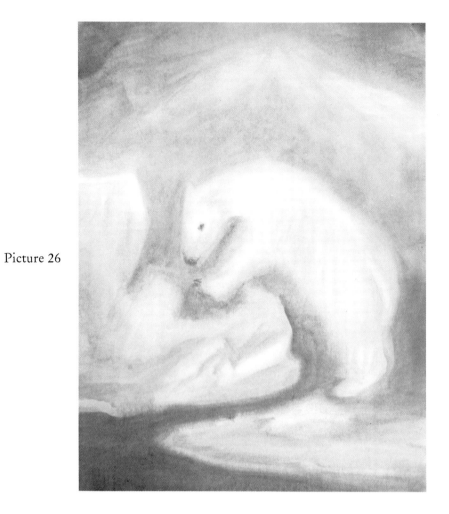

Picture 26

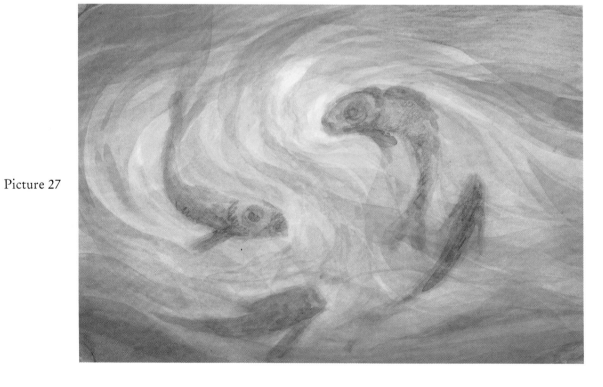

Picture 27

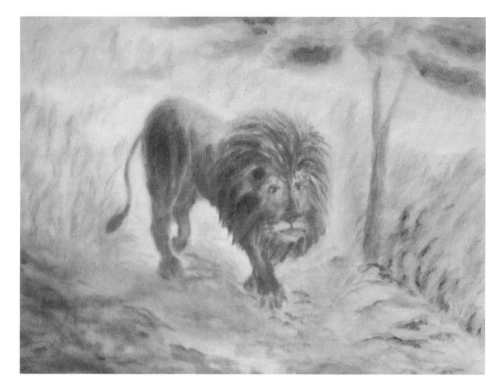

Picture 28

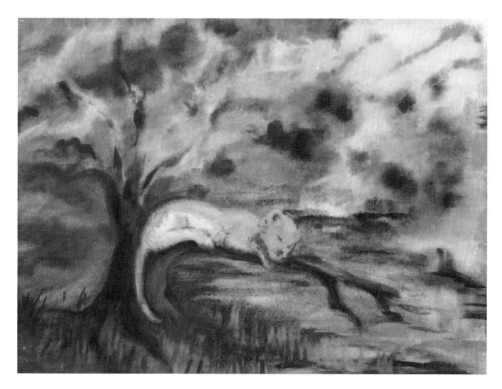

Picture 29

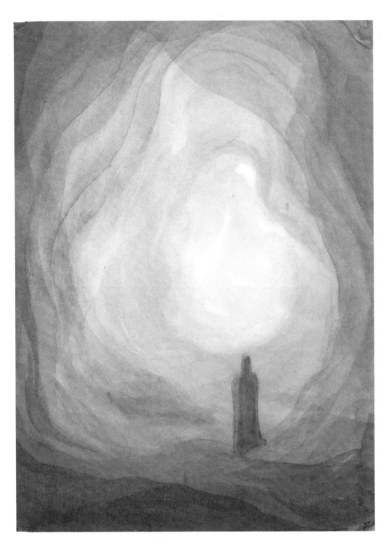

Picture 30

Picture 31

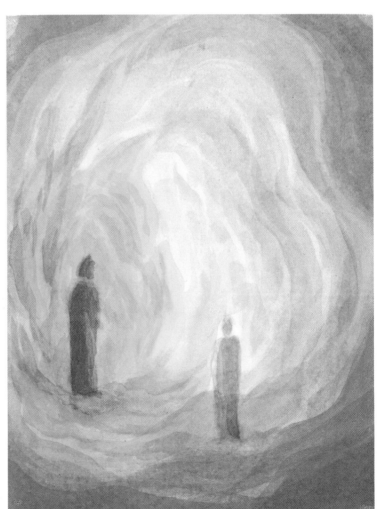

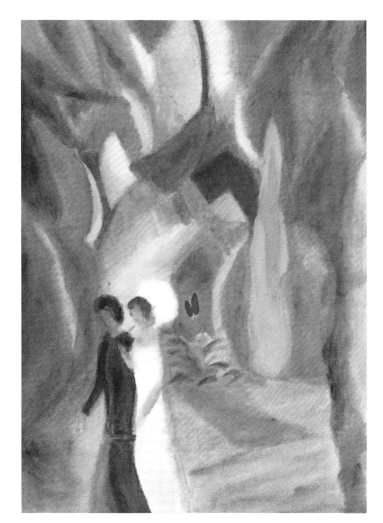

Picture 32

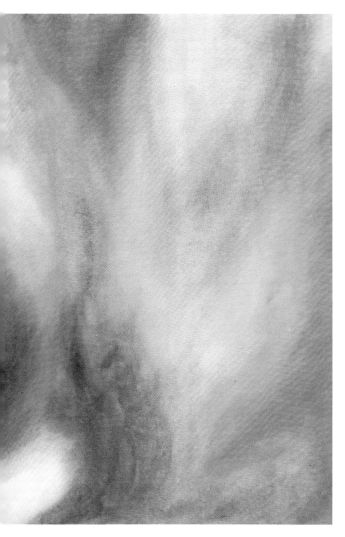

Picture 33

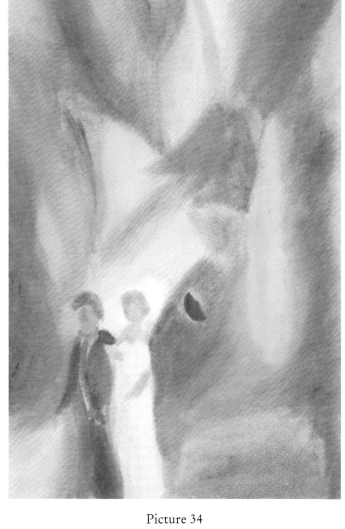

Picture 34

Picture 35

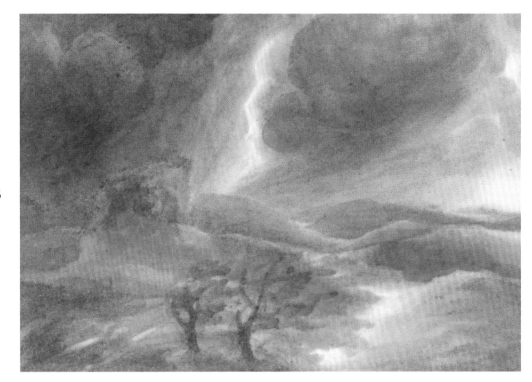

Picture 36

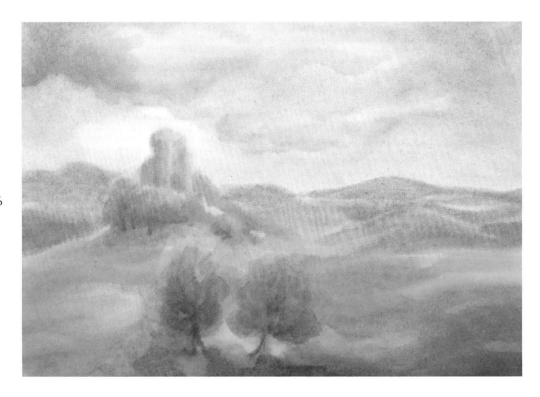

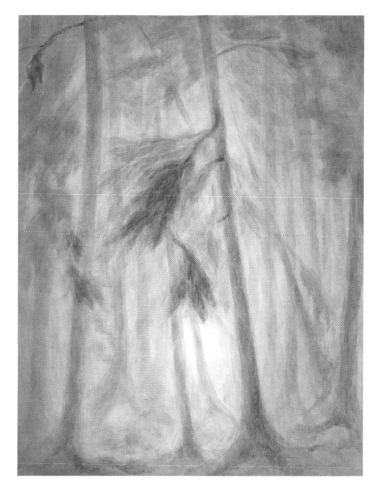

Picture 37

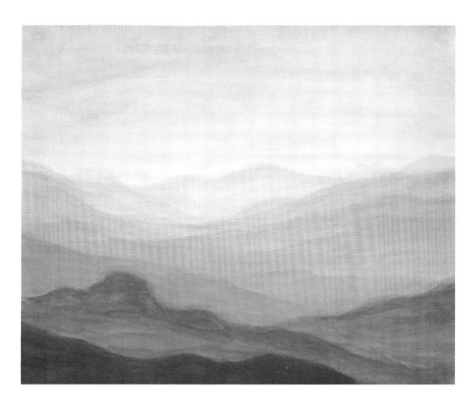

Picture 38

Picture 39

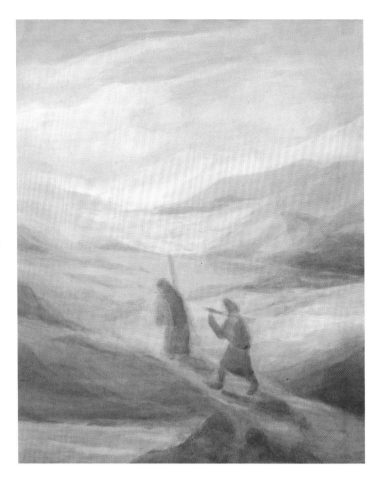

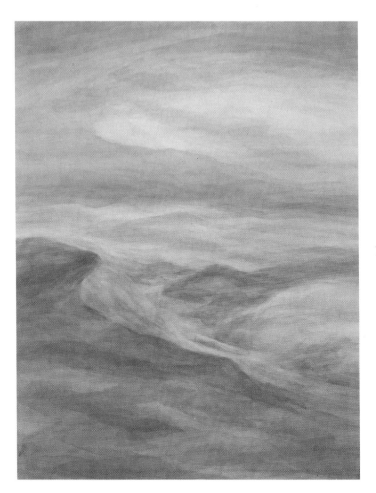

Picture 40

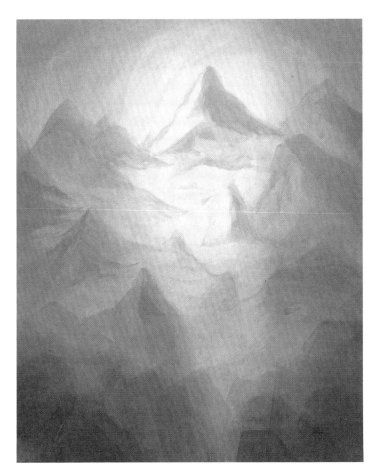

Picture 41

Picture 42

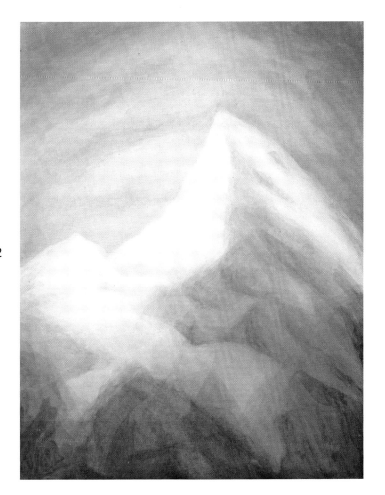

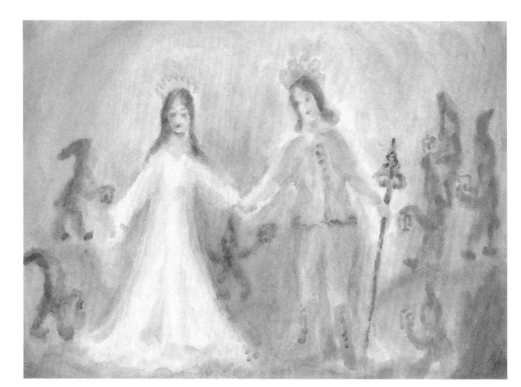

Picture 43

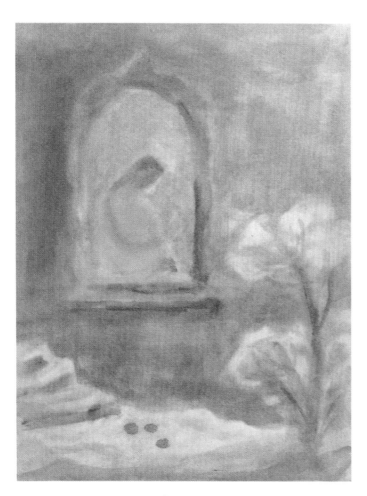

Picture 44

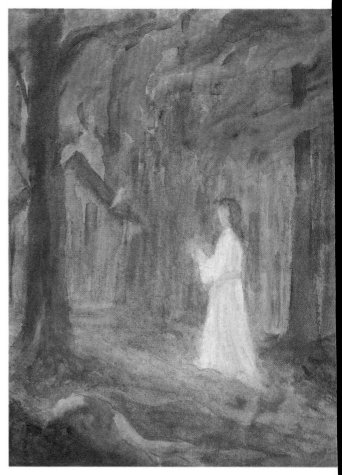

Picture 45

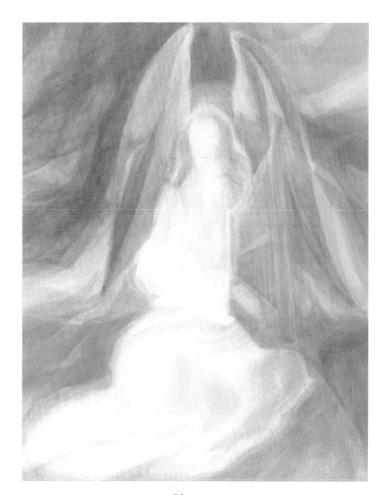

Picture 46

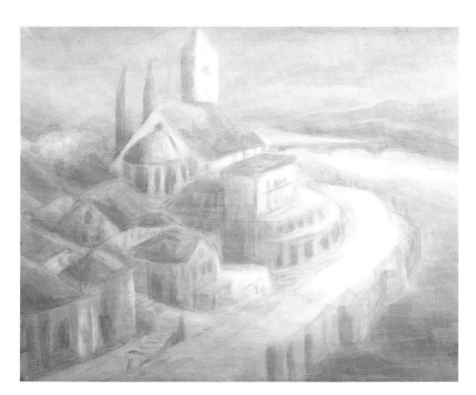

Picture 47

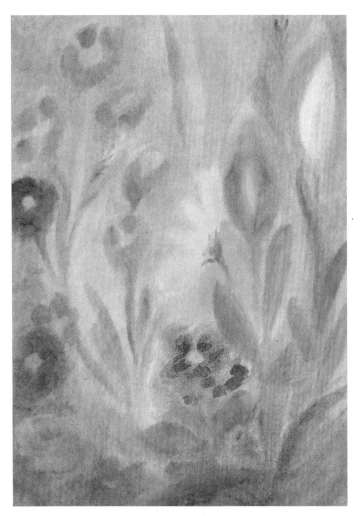

Picture 48

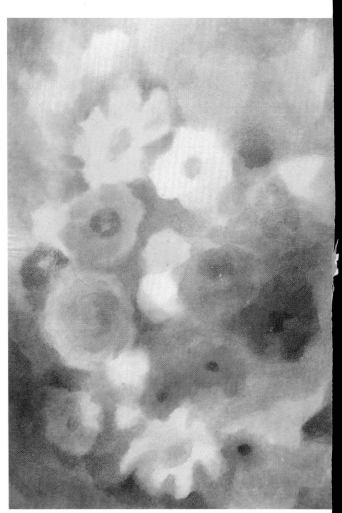

Picture 49

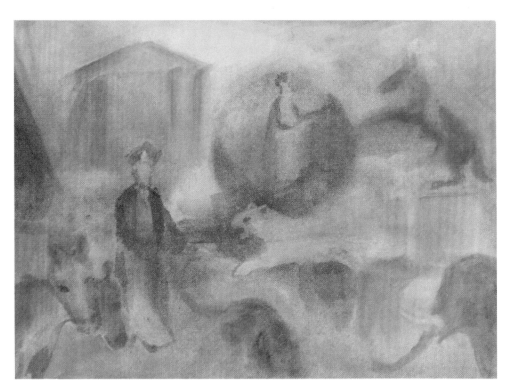

Picture 50